Ageless

Ageless

A yogi's secrets to a long and
healthy life

R. Sharath Jois

with

Isha Singh Sawhney

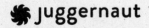

JUGGERNAUT BOOKS

KS House, 118 Shahpur Jat, New Delhi 110049, India

First published by Juggernaut Books 2018

ISBN 9788193876787

Typeset in Adobe Caslon Pro by R. Ajith Kumar, Noida

Printed at Manipal Technologies Limited, Manipal

To my grandfather,
who gave me this practice

Contents

Introduction

From sickness to health

As a child, I was always ill. My early years were racked with pain. Tonsillitis, rheumatic fever and infections from the fever, hernia . . . you name it, I had it. I was so sick that the doctors forbade me from riding a cycle, which, you can imagine, is quite devastating for a child. My dreams of becoming a professional cricketer were also dashed because my sickness didn't allow me to register for the National Cadet Corps. I spent months in bed, convalescing from illnesses. I was a miserable pre-teen desperate to be outdoors playing with other children.

But there was one silver lining.

My time spent in bed meant I watched a lot of movies! Especially *Ramayana*. Rama, Arjuna, Ganesha and Bhima were the superheroes of our time. They were intelligent, strong and blessed with supernatural powers. But my personal favourite was Hanuman. I probably watched *Sampoorna Ramayan* about twenty times as a child.

I loved Hanuman's spirituality, his power and his devotion to Rama. Hanuman is so humble, he doesn't even understand how immense his strength is until Jambavan the bear tells him about his capabilities and encourages him to fly to Lanka in search of Sita.

As a sickly child, I wanted to be just like Hanuman – strong and spiritual. He was my superhero. Perhaps I was too young to realize that my biggest strength was with me in my home – my grandfather, Pattabhi Jois.

I was born on 29 September 1971 in Mysore. During the early years of my childhood, my mother, sister and I lived with my father in Jamshedpur, Jharkhand. We would often visit my maternal grandparents in Mysore. At the time, my grandfather, Pattabhi Jois, taught Ashtanga Yoga in the tradition of T. Krishnamacharya to Indian students and a handful of foreigners.

Pattabhi Jois's father, my great-grandfather, had been an astrologer, priest and landholder, and by the time my grandfather was five years old he had been instructed in Sanskrit and Hindu rituals, as all Brahmin boys were. In 1927, my grandfather – along with B.K.S. Iyengar and Indra Devi, under the mentorship of the then king of Mysore, Krishna Raja Wadiyar IV, also known as the philosopher king – started studying with T. Krishnamacharya.

In 1948, Guruji started the Ashtanga Yoga Research Institute in Lakshmipuram with the aim of experimenting with the curative aspects of yoga as taught to him by Krishnamacharya, whose main source was the famous *Yoga Korunta* – the ancient manuscript of Ashtanga Yoga attributed to the sage Vamana. No one has seen a copy of the *Yoga Korunta* and there are doubts that it existed as its teachings were passed on by word of mouth to T. Krishnamacharya. But it has unrefutably inspired one of the most powerful and beautiful yoga systems that has spread rapidly around the world in the last few decades.

In 1975, when I was four, we moved back to Mysore as my father was not around much because of his job and I had a very bad bout of tonsillitis which could be best treated in a bigger city. The illness compromised my immunity further. Later, when I turned eleven, I was diagnosed with a rare illness called rheumatic fever, which can take anywhere from five to ten years of antibiotic medication to heal completely. I was physically depleted from all these illnesses.

Once we moved to Mysore, I, along with the children of other students, started yoga with my grandfather. At that time, his two sons, Manju and Ramesh, were also studying with him, assisting him as he taught. And my mother, having also studied with him at a very young age, was also teaching on her own merit. Yoga had always been deeply ingrained in our family.

Yoga with my grandfather changed my health for the better. Instead of a decade of antibiotics, a series of very simple postures helped me become stronger. I could feel my body heal and repair. As my immunity grew, I started stepping out of the house more. I found I had more energy to play with the children in our neighbourhood. The doctors said my recovery was a miracle because of how severely my young body had been weakened by the onslaught of illnesses. Later, I would learn that the 'miracle' was not mystical; it was simply the result of the practical and logical yogic practice to which my grandfather introduced me.

The benefits of a yogic practice and lifestyle are, of course, difficult to explain to a child, and perhaps even to most adults. Later, when I was stronger, my formal tutelage began, and it was against my will. As a youngster, I resented being made to practise yoga. Like other adolescent boys, I wanted to be left alone to play cricket all day long. My love for cricket has remained. Even today my son and I never miss a single cricket match on television.

Every day after school, my grandfather (soon to become my Guruji, I just didn't know it then) would make my sister and me practise with him at his shala, then at his home in Lakshmipuram. My friends who'd be playing cricket outside on the streets would ask for me, but my grandfather would sternly turn them away. We were all frightened of him because he was very strict. So, when he left the room to have coffee in the kitchen, I would sneak out of the back door to play cricket on the street. You see, my friends had a vested interest in me because I was a very good batsman. After his coffee break, my grandfather, upon realizing his pupil was missing, would waste no time in coming to look for me. And the great Pattabhi Jois would open the doors of our house and holler down the streets of Lakshmipuram, furiously calling my name. My friends would tell me to hide. And I would! I'd find a good spot in the gullies around our house, only to emerge after my grandfather had given up his search. Later he would chide me, 'People come from all over to practise here and our own children are wasting the opportunity…' I was extremely scared of him, but the fear did not stop me from being errant. Such is the power of youth!

I learned the yogic way of life from my grandfather

Few people know this, but my grandfather would wake up every day at 4 a.m. and do his morning chants, while making coffee for everyone in the house. No matter who you were you would get coffee made by him in your bed! What a luxury! He was a very disciplined man. Even on a holiday he would give everyone coffee in bed! He always washed his own clothes, even when he was eighty-five.

He lived a very simple life. He never socialized. Yet he didn't force any of this on me. I never thought I would go back to yoga. Or become a teacher. He never expected me to come to the shala at four every morning. He never imposed rules or regulations on me. But he was so inspirational, I followed in his footsteps without any questions.

The only place he would correct me was in the shala. There I was just another student. He gave me no special treatment. He pushed me more, in fact! The way we learn and teach in India is so powerful. We don't pamper our children or our students. There was extra pressure on me to work hard. I liked to think of it as encouragement in disguise. He would get very angry with me in the shala when I didn't perform. I was scolded in front of everyone.

My quiet and wondrous transformation

Despite my early rebellions, yoga was deeply entrenched in my life and my daily routine. I would practise every evening after school. Back then, I was just playing with asanas. My body was very supple, and it was easy for me to do the postures. I was simply having fun. I was not concentrating on my breath or anything. It's amazing that such little effort helped me get over the illness and weakness that had caught hold of my body.

In 1989, I was seventeen years old when I had my first experience teaching Ashtanga Yoga. My mother, Saraswati, had gone to the US and my sister and I oversaw her students and her shala for four months. I only had to help a few students – mostly ladies from the neighbourhood who had been coming to my mother for years for a little exercise. But I hated teaching there. All the ladies wanted to do was gossip and chat! And all I wanted was to go out and meet my friends. I waited impatiently for those four months to get over. But, when I look back now, I realize how valuable that experience of assisting was to me as a yoga teacher.

Two years later, at nineteen, I started assisting my grandfather, who was getting along in years, at his shala. When I started the second time around, my once strict grandfather had softened. He had lost one son, Ramesh, and the other, Manju, had moved to the US permanently. I was doing a diploma in computers and had a year left to complete the course. So, I started helping him and did a little of my own practice too. Unknown to me, something was slowly shifting within me.

Ashtanga Yoga works in quiet ways.

'*Purvabhyasena tenaiva hriyate hyavasho'pi sah*,' says the Bhagavad Gita. This means – in this birth the mind will be attracted to yoga by tendencies developed towards yoga in previous births.

The eight limbs of Ashtanga, as outlined by Patanjali in the Yoga Sutras, work towards internal and external purification that help you connect with the Universal Self or atman. Through this practice, whatever your reason for starting may be, results will show – if I may use the cliché – slowly, but surely.

As I became serious about Ashtanga Yoga, I realized this had to become my sadhana (a disciplined and dedicated study). I was no longer simply Ashtanga. During those months, something marvellous happened both inside and around me. I had been watching people come and go, learning, being helped by yoga, and then an inexplicable transformation happened in my own practice.

In the beginning it is tough to learn a new skill or art. After a certain stage you start to enjoy that pressure, those challenges and the process. And when you understand the system – the pressure falls away. As I understood breathing and asana and vinyasa, advancements happened.

The asana part of Ashtanga is extremely challenging. But to experience many asanas and to advance yourself, you have to go through all those difficulties. In my life I have learned many postures. I had the time, I had the passion, I had the best Ashtanga teacher, and even then I found it very challenging.

But I wanted to go deep into the practice. When you want to go deeper, just like when you reach deep into a jungle, you are bound to face many challenges. The important thing is to remember that this is temporary, and you will emerge on the other side stronger.

In *Yoga Mala*, my grandfather writes, as the weak and sick practise yoga or perform certain asanas specific to their ailments, under the guidance of their guru, their strength increases while disease and weaknesses get eliminated. Many incurable diseases, including mental illnesses and leprosy, have been cured through the practice of yoga, leaving even physicians dumbfounded. I later realized that it was yoga and the principles of yogic living that had nurtured me back to good health as a child.

In 1997, my grandmother passed away. I had been her favourite grandchild. Her advice and support were the foundations on which my practice was formed. When I got a job at an electronics company, she advised me not to go to Bangalore and to instead commit myself to my grandfather. As I became increasingly more serious about my practice, she would feed me twice a day. She would mix sambar and rice and put it in my hand. This is a very traditional way of eating called tuttuanna that shows the affection between mother and child. She made sure I got all the nutrition I needed. And of course, all the love. My grandmother was a strong woman with a great sense of humour. She emanated a warmth that attracted people – from yoga students to government officials, elderly people to children who would drop in for a chat and her special coffee; the best coffee in all of Mysore!

The 1990s were generous to my spiritual journey

and my yogic education. There were very few students with my grandfather at the time, out of which fewer than twenty were foreigners. I practised for three hours every day and felt the immense pain of my body changing. From that change first came stability. I saw how within my body, with the practise of vinyasa – the act of breathing and moving while practising an asana – a purification was taking place. As my blood became hot, it became cleansed and started to circulate freely; it rid my body of toxins, impurities and disease, and then it became easy for me to purify my nervous system. And through all this came stability of my mind.

How Ashtanga and I grew

In December 1997, after having been denied a visa thrice, I finally travelled abroad for the first time, to Sydney. Soon after that, my grandfather and I visited the US a few times. Around this time yoga, and Ashtanga Yoga specifically, started gaining popularity at a phenomenal pace. Hollywood celebrities like Gwyneth Paltrow and Willem Dafoe were doing Ashtanga regularly and had become staunch advocates of the method. Paltrow practised with Guruji when we visited New York in the aftermath of 9/11. At this time in American history, Ashtanga became a release and a powerful healer for Americans.

As its popularity grew, the number of students coming to the shala in Mysore also increased. After Americans came Europeans, then Japanese and Chinese. Yoga began to spread like wildfire. I did demos from Japan to Chile. My grandfather would do the counts and I would do the postures. In 2000, I visited the US for a demo. People had no idea where yoga came from. In Japan, people thought yoga came from America!

And so I had to explain. Yoga is Bharat Bhumi. Just one look at Indian history and you will see how even before India was India, people came here from all over the world to learn yoga.

Today, students and shalas of K. Pattabhi Jois Ashtanga Yoga Institute (KPJAYI) are spread over more than a hundred countries.

Evam paramparā prāptam imam rājarsayo viduh |
Sa kāleneha mahatā yogo nastah parantapa ||[1]

O scorcher of foes! This Yoga handed down from teacher to disciple in succession, was known to the Rājarsis (royal sages). But owing to long lapse of time, it was lost to the world.

The eight limbs of Ashtanga

Guruji lost both his sons. He missed them. I think I came to fill this gap in his life, and in my grandmother's. I was a support to him. And we became very close. We would go everywhere together. And his passion for philosophy would follow us everywhere. This was the privilege of being his grandson. We would talk a lot about Shankaracharya or the Gita or Upanishads. This was the special part of our relationship. As a teacher, he expected his students to respond to his passions, which ranged from philosophy to asanas. He saw this interest in me and showed me books and talked to me about different topics. When you seek and are curious, your teacher sees it and tries to give you as much as possible. Even outside the classroom, we would have long chats about philosophy. He would quote stories and sometimes when he forgot a verse my grandmother would back him up!

Literally translated, Ashtanga means: ash – eight and tanga – limbed. Derived from Patanjali's Yoga Sutra, this defines the path to discovery of the Universal Self or atma through the practice and adherence of these eight steps:

1. Yama: moral discipline
2. Niyama: observances

3. Asana: physical posture
4. Pranayama: breath control
5. Pratyahara: sense withdrawal
6. Dharana: concentration
7. Dhyana: absorption or meditation
8. Samadhi: absorption into the Universal or enlightenment

The way to make the mind one-pointed, says Guruji in *Yoga Mala*, in order to see the Universal Self, is to follow these steps. These limbs are just as important, or more, as a yogi's physical asana practice. To develop a spiritual practice, it's important to be aware of these limbs, otherwise your yoga is meaningless. Let's look at the first two limbs, yama and niyama, as they concern and can be adopted by everyone.

Yama refers to a universal moral code that applies to everyone. They are a guide to yogic living. Yamas are:

Satya: truthfulness
Ahimsa: non-violence
Asteya: non-stealing
Aparigraha: non-possessiveness
Brahmacharya: fidelity or celibacy

Niyamas, or observances, are recommended habits for a long and healthy life. They are personal practices which are, once again, for everyone no matter what your situation is. Niyamas include:

Saucha: cleanliness
Santosa: contentment
Tapas: self-discipline
Svadhaya: self-study
Iswara pranidhana: surrender to God

Together these provide an infallible moral value system and practical daily guideline for us within any given context. And while these are important concepts for non-yogis too, we must not forget that it becomes easier to dedicate oneself to these limbs with a strong asana practice.

During discussions on the Bhagavad Gita, Guruji would often talk about the sixteen chapters that explore the yogic method and what your mental state should be both on and off the mat. In this book, I mention the Gita many times. Don't get me wrong. I'm not pushing a particular religious agenda. The Bhagavad Gita does not belong to any one religion, nor does it talk to the people of just one religion. It belongs to all humanity. It addresses all human beings. In the

Bhagavad Gita, Lord Krishna talks about philosophies and how to conduct yourself, what your karma is, what your duties should be. And every single message in it is applicable to any human being across every religion, whether you are a yoga practitioner or not.

Why yogis live long lives

Tirumalai Krishnamacharya lived till 100. Pattabhi Jois lived till ninety-three. B.K.S. Iyengar lived till ninety-six. They were all serious yoga practitioners with a big following.

What was the secret of their long lives?

In *Yoga Mala,* Guruji talks of the yoga practitioner who can achieve anything in the world by a dedicated practice of the limbs of yoga. Such a practitioner can even redo creation, as Sage Vishvamitra did when he created another Indraloka – world of the gods – for 'a lower-caste man' who wanted to go to heaven, making the gods fearful of his strength.

One's journey to immortality begins with a strong body. Your body is the home you live in. Without a strong foundation, your house will crumble. Of course, you also need a steady spiritual base.

That is why yogis live long, healthy lives. They dedicate themselves to clean and simple practices and routines that make them strong and ageless. Yogis live long lives because they have built strong foundations for themselves. The bedrock of which is minimalism – less is always more simplicity – happiness, discipline, empathy and selflessness. These are values that have been forgotten by the modern world. The best part is that all of these values are free. It just takes a change of perspective to achieve them.

Today, a purification through Hatha Yoga means first developing an asana practice. Yogis live long, healthy lives (never forget it's not just quantity, it is also quality) because there is an inherent focus on living, eating, sleeping, walking and reacting *mindfully*.

Of course, a disciplined yoga practice is just the first step. Yoga helps you listen to and strengthen your body. But in due time, it also makes you sensitive to other aspects of life – that connect you with other people and humanity.

Another reason why yogis live to a hundred years is that they keep things simple! They eat sattvic foods which have for centuries been known to keep the mind and body light and clean. They understand maya and its trappings.

Today, more than ever before, life comes with anxieties not simply of everyday routine, but also those fostered by the media. Yogis are constantly bombarded with what/how/where/when to eat/wear/sleep/work. I, for one, yearn for those days when the only advice we got was passed down undiluted and full of anecdotes from parent to child. In a life surrounded by toxins, we desperately need to find a way to conquer those toxins of the mind, our senses and our bodies. We need to take notes from simpler times on how to uncomplicate our lives.

All of this is also connected to the mind. A healthy body needs to be complemented with strong emotional and mental well-being. Today, our minds are brittle, fragile, overwhelmed because we have stopped taking care. Our minds need tending to, just like any other organ. In an age rife with depression and medications, yogis can provide a prototype for dealing with emotional stress of modern-day life and help find a space of quietude, confidence and peace. And when the mind is at peace, we will automatically see a reduction in lifestyle diseases that are so prevalent today. There is no magic here. You only need to look on the internet to find all the studies corroborating the connections between mind and body health.

If nothing else, take inspiration from my story. I went from being a very ill child to a yoga guru, who teaches thousands of students every year. It was my yogic life and practice that enabled me to become who I am today. And that is the beauty of yoga. Everyone can be healthy and fit by learning from the lives of yogis. I hope my story can show you how yoga and yogic living have helped me overcome the challenges that life threw in my direction. Now, you too can benefit from them. It doesn't matter if you are young, old, sick, frail, thin, fat, shy, inflexible – yoga has the solution to all problems.

Through this book I will show you how yogic practices related to eating, breathing, asana and seva can contribute positively to your mental and physical health. I have tried to present simple ideas that are not intimidating – from walking barefoot to connect with the earth to eating fewer times in the day. These ideas may contradict recommendations, such as eating six meals, that you may have heard all your life, but they have come to us from ancient Vedic texts and we can't disregard their wisdom.

Remember, living like a yogi does not mean renouncing the world. To be a yogi, you don't have to give up your life in the city and run off to the mountains. I am not asking you to do any such thing. This book aims to make adopting the habits of a yogi as easy and commonplace as brushing one's teeth.

Living like a yogi is about becoming connected with vitality and health. It's about spending time under a tree, reading a book, breathing in as much fresh air as one can, being kind to other living beings, ahimsa, and giving without thinking of taking back. With so much conflict in the world, and the onslaught of 24/7 news and the culture of the internet, it's more important than ever to turn our gaze towards yoga, and go back to the principles of yogic living to achieve peace and strength of character.

If by eating correctly, living consciously, breathing deeply and doing basic asanas we can alleviate chronic lifestyle-related pain and discomfort, then why should we all not have a little bit of yoga in our lives, in a form that is easy to digest?

Outside of daily habits, I have also put together a basic asana routine accessible to all people, even those who are not yet ritualized into a regular practice. As they say in the Yoga Sutra,

Sa tu dīrghakāla nairantarya satkārādarāsevito drdhabhūmih ||[2]

Practice becomes firmly grounded when it has been cultivated for a long time uninterruptedly with earnest devotion.

Introduction

Yoga should be a part of everyone's life, no matter what religion you follow. We are all human beings first. A yogic life can help us lead a healthy, stress- and delusion-free life. It can alleviate the suffering of the mind and the body. I want to demystify a yogi's life, while also releasing it from the Westernized, commercial aspects it has become synonymous with. I hope this book can motivate people to do some basic yoga and unlock the secrets to living a long, healthy and peaceful life.

~

- Simple practices and routines can make us strong and ageless.
- Develop a spiritual practice, otherwise your yoga is meaningless.
- Eat small, eat local and eat at noon, when your jathra agani is at its peak.

1

Eat Less to Live Longer

In a land far, far away, in a time long, long ago, a five-year-old boy is not allowed to sit on his father King Uttanapada's lap. Angered, the boy, Prince Dhruva, leaves for the forest to look for God, and childishly demands from Lord Vishnu a kingdom bigger than his father's.

The child prince starts an intense meditation. He doesn't eat for days, then eats only leaves and grass, drinks water only every nine days. By the fourth month, he suspends his breath and stands only on one leg. The demigods are worried. At one point, Dhruva's suspension of breath is so powerful, the whole world stops breathing. When Lord Vishnu goes down to meet his devotee, Dhruva realizes how materialistic and immature his demands were. He promises to devote his life to God, but Lord Vishnu in his infinite wisdom blesses him. Dhruva goes on to rule the earth for 36,000 years in a fair, kind and just manner.

Dhruva's story (this particular one is from the Bhagavata Purana) is just one of many in our scriptures that address why fasting is and was so important to ascetics or those trying to achieve a higher spiritual connection.

Fasts help achieve siddhi (psychic power) that leads to haadi vidya; a knowledge, upon acquiring which, one feels neither hunger nor thirst and can go without food or water for several days at a stretch. Without these distractions, one can concentrate on one's tapasya or quest to connect with the Universal Self. Often in the epics, sages and kings would devote themselves to great penance to achieve their goals, and abstinence from food was considered the highest of sacrifices, because subsisting on prana, awakens the life force within. Quite simply put, prana is the Sanskrit word for life force.

But don't get me wrong. I'm not asking you to starve yourself.

Of course, these fantastical stories seem absurd and impractical today. But we should not relegate them to the realm of mythology either, because they hold a secret to longevity we've all forgotten – frugality. And the first aspect of our modern lives that we seem incapable of applying this secret to is eating.

Today, food is immensely abundant. Food (especially junk and processed food) is cheap and found everywhere at the press of a button. Yet this very abundance is making us sicker. It causes us pain. Obesity rates and heart diseases are at their highest ever in history. And food lies at the centre of most illnesses. The very same substances which give us life are killing us now. The father of Ayurveda, Charaka says, 'Even food, which is the life of living creatures, if taken in an improper manner destroys life.'[1]

We've not only forgotten frugality, we've abandoned it altogether. So, in this chapter I'm going to make a case for why eating less can change your life dramatically.

~

Since longevity is difficult to study in human beings, independent studies were conducted in the 1980s by the University of Wisconsin and the National Institute of Aging in Maryland in the United States of America on rhesus monkeys – the closest animals to human beings in similarities of ageing and age-related disease and decay. Nutritionists observed that monkeys put on calorie-restrictive diets showed a marked delay in ageing and the onset of age-related disease. Less food meant longer lives.

Eating less, as advocated by yogis, has been scientifically proven to reverse ageing. Undereating, as the theory goes, slows down the body's metabolism in a way such that it produces less damaging oxidants – agents that rust the body from within. When your body isn't working hard to digest food from the last meal you ate, you are giving necessary biological repairs a chance to take place. Makes sense, doesn't it?

Neither my grandfather nor Krishnamacharya read these reports, but throughout their lives, their diets were simple and restricted. And they both lived long and healthy lives. My grandfather died when he was 93 years old, while Krishnamacharya lived till a 100. Until my grandfather died in May 2009, he was very active and taught almost to the very end.

There is more and more proof in the assertion that eating less is one of the secrets to a long life. Yogis have practised this for many years. Eating less, combined with the other food habits I discuss later in the book, can help add not just years to your life, but nourished, healthy years. But first let's take a look at what yogis think and say about digestion.

The fire in your belly

It's only now that modern science has begun to understand the importance a healthy gut plays in the well-being of an organism. But ancient yogis and vaidyas were on to it long before modern science.

Fire in Vedic times was the great cleanser and purifier. It linked the mortal world to the divine. To appease the gods, one made sacrifices to fire. The significance of fire sacrifices was not lost on the Ayurvedic tradition. But here, sacrifice was thought of differently. Sacrifice was an internal offering. The one we made with food. Ayurveda considers eating a kind of daily inner sacrifice because the region of your stomach is dominated by the fire element. This potent fire of digestion, called Jathragni, was the seat of all physical balance and harmony. Jathragni, according to Ayurveda, is how your food gets digested. It is the act of digestion in your digestive tract.[2]

If this doesn't make sense to you – think about it like this. Food is fuel. Without it, there will be no life. If the stomach is where this fuel gets transformed into energy, then there must be some kind of combustion taking place. And combustion requires fire. So the vaidyas imagined the stomach to be a great sacrificial fire that ensures our existence. Hence, the act of eating was considered a pure and crucial inner sacrifice. Eating is considered 'sacrificial worship' and an Ayurvedic text goes so far as to call any person who eats in a healthy manner a 'fire worshipper'.

If you've ever built a fire or seen someone doing it, you'll know that fire needs a good balance of fuel and air to light up properly. Give it soggy wood and it will not kindle. Pile it up with too much wood and there will still be no fire. This goes for the fire in our stomachs too. Load it with too much food, and it will extinguish combustion. Give it nothing, it will corrode the intestinal lining and stomach with its gastric acids. Eating, then, becomes a fine craft of stoking this wondrous fire. Today, most people are guilty of overfeeding this digestive fire and hence suffer from a host of digestive issues. With such an abundance of food, we desperately need to reassess quantities. Yogis understand this ancient science and hence rarely fall sick.

You will initially find it difficult to eat less. But think for a minute of your body as a machine. If you load your 10 kg washing machine with 15 kg of clothes it is bound to work slowly and eventually break down at some point. And because our bodies are extraordinary machines you can't overload them with too much food. If you overfeed your body, you will damage it because essentially you are killing the digestive fire. Everything you put inside your body will be processed, broken down and assimilated. And this background work that we don't see requires time. It takes five to six hours for your body to digest what you put into it in the form of food, so it's very important to limit what you eat.

Let's now look at what it means to have a healthy digestive constitution and how much food is required for our optimum function.

Eating less results in a healthy constitution

Have you ever wondered why some people are hyperactive and some inherently slow? Why some body types are prone to quick weight loss and gain and some never put on weight, no matter how many pieces of rava fried fish or samosas they eat? Some get angry in a heartbeat, while others stew in their juices for days and months and then slowly explode? Or why some of us grey prematurely, and others go bald?

None of the above is random.

Ayurveda describes all of our individual idiosyncrasies and characteristics according to our doshas. What this means is that each one of us has a unique blueprint that defines us. According to

Ayurveda, these blueprints are scripted by the five elements – earth, fire, water, air and ether. All these elements are present in us. The word 'dosha' comes from the word 'dosh' meaning fault. Doshas are the by-product of an organism being alive. There are three main doshas – vata, kapha and pitta. And these are present in all living beings, mostly in combination.

Vata is represented by wind and ether. It is a moody artist, responsible for all motion, ideas, dreams and movement. Vata is kinetic energy, quick, light and always raring to go. Pitta, on the other hand, is potential energy. A creation of water and fire, it takes care of all transformations in the body. Hence, digestion, cognitive ability, the processing and assimilation of information are its domains. Pitta is the pinprick of life in your eyes. Kapha is made of water and earth, and it governs the areas of stability and lubrication so that the whole show runs smoothly.

A healthy constitution is when the three doshas are in harmony. However, if there is excess, lack or impurity in our lives, then an error manifests, upsetting the balance of the doshas. This is when illness rears its head and the body is thrown into chaos. Eating incorrectly is the surest way of doing this. In the digestive system, excess vata means flatulence and constipation. Too much pitta leads to acidity and excessive hunger. And excess kapha means indigestion. We need to feed the digestive fire the good stuff and, most relevant today, in the right quantities.

Today, most of us eat too much and too often, and so we are in effect dousing the fire and are beset with a host of digestive problems. From obesity to flatulence, haemorrhoids to cancers, the list is endless. But all of this can be cured if we are mindful about our food intake.

It's hard to change what we eat in one day. Switching to a completely new healthy diet takes effort, time and also money. But how about quantity? That's not very difficult if we think about it. We don't have to buy new ingredients or equipment. We just need to reduce the amount we eat.

Less food makes a sharper mind

Yogis wake up early for their practice. If we eat too much, our bodies become sluggish and heavy. If our stomachs are too full, we can't concentrate. Yogis usually eat one big meal, and then something light in the evenings. According to the shastras and the Bhagavad Gita, as long as your yoga doesn't suffer, you should limit your food, your sleep and karma. Here, think of karma as your daily work and routine or any action in your daily life. And just like anything else, you cannot work for long periods of time with no rest. You must experience other things in life.

Try to apply this principle to your life. Watch how you perform at a meeting after a big meal and how you fare after a smaller one. Is it easier to read or work when your stomach is stuffed with food or when it is lighter? I think you already know the answers to these questions.

Overeating disturbs the body, makes you physically and mentally sleepy and inactive. To keep your mind sharp, eat foods with a low glycaemic index (GI), which allow the sugars in foods to be processed and broken down more steadily. It's like going up an escalator instead of a lift. Foods that come in packets or are processed work quickly, send a burst of energy in your body. To see this in action, observe a child after he/she has eaten a chocolate. The child will go from inactive to dizzyingly active in no time! This is the effect of simple sugars. Once our bodies, much like a child, get addicted to those quick bursts of energy, it's more likely to trick you into craving these efficient sugar rushes. And that's why most of us reach out for a biscuit and tea in the afternoon.

Whereas foods like oats, non-starchy vegetables (such as cauliflower, carrots, cucumber, spinach, eggplant, etc.) and whole wheat breads break down and release their energies more gradually, thus, making you less likely to crave a quick sugar rush.

Do not eat breakfast like a king

Yuktāhāra vihārasya yukta cestasya karmasu |
Yukta svapnāvabodhasya yogo bhavati duhkhahā ||[3]

For one who is temperate in food and recreation, who is detached and self-restrained in work, who is regulated in sleep and in vigil – yoga brings about the cessation of the travails of samsara.

These lines from the Bhagavad Gita ask us to keep everything in balance, never overindulging in sleep, food, work or recreation. It suggests that if your life is balanced, your mind will be balanced too.

My grandfather and T. Krishnamacharya followed this dictum seriously. They lived meagrely, following the middle path. And that was the biggest secret to their long and healthy lives.

My grandfather never ate breakfast. At night, Guruji avoided most foods, and would eat just a banana and drink a big glass of milk. Both Guruji and Krishnamacharya drank a lot of milk, morning and evening. It was only when he turned eighty-five that he began to eat a small breakfast, because he would get tired. Krishnamacharya too, like my grandfather, would not eat breakfast.

We've always been told to eat 'breakfast like a king'. But how many of us have stopped to think about this old adage? Eating a heavy breakfast may not always be conducive to productivity. Your brain is most active in the morning. Eating a light breakfast or skipping it altogether will make you feel light and keep you on your toes, whereas eating a heavy meal first thing in the morning will make you feel lethargic and tired, because your body will expend all its energy on digesting that big meal. And so contrary to popular opinion, you don't need to eat like a king before you start your day. At the most, you need just a little energy to set you off. If you have gastric issues or simply need some energy, eat a light, nutritious meal of fruits or sprouts.

When I am teaching in Mysore, I wake up at 1 a.m. to finish my own yoga practice. An Ashtanga practitioner needs to start at this sacred hour – a time when the mind is quiet and receptive. For years I would eat nothing until lunch, subsisting only on coffee. In fact, I would often say 'no coffee, no prana' because it was the only way I could wake up to teach! But this habit started giving me painful acid reflux, so now I eat a bowl of oats with nuts, seeds and a sprinkle of spices after I finish my morning practice. It's important to find your own equation.

Eating less or nothing in the morning may take some getting used to. Try it one day and monitor how your body feels. You may get hunger pangs, but that is because you are used to feeding your body a lot of food. So, it will be unhappy and demanding when you take that away, just as a cigarette smoker gets withdrawal pangs when he/she is deprived of nicotine. But if you persist, you will find that you can think better, your mind will be sharper and you will feel less sleepy and lazy and as a result be more productive through the first half of the morning.

That being said, do check with your doctor before embarking on any dietary changes.

Eat one big meal a day, and make that lunch

In my home lunch is the biggest meal of the day. It traditionally consists of rice and sambar and fresh salad. Sometimes we replace rice with ragi mudde or ragi balls. Ragi mudde, the food of farmers in

Karnataka, are just dough balls of millet cooked and then eaten with sambar or rasam. But they are packed with nutrition.

The logic behind making lunch your biggest meal is really quite simple – you have the rest of the day to digest it.[4] Also, according to Ayurveda, the body's jathra agni is at its peak at noon, when the sun is at its strongest. This is the time the body's pitta, the dosha responsible for transformations, is most active, making it easiest for food to be assimilated with no side effects like acidity or heartburn.

However, eating a large meal is not an excuse to eat anything you want. Your plate must have a mix of complex carbohydrates, proteins, fibre, and a healthy amount of green leafy vegetables that are your source of vitamins and minerals. For lunch, look for foods that are packed with both nutrition and energy. Replace the simple sugars of white rice that lead to that dreadful afternoon drowsiness with finger millets or whole grains like amaranth and quinoa, which take longer to digest. Millets are a healthy choice for people suffering from diabetes as they have a low glycaemic index and are rich in antioxidants.

A large bowl of salad with finger millets or whole grains, protein in the form of tofu or animal protein and boiled sprouts is excellent for those who want a change from their dal–sabzi routine. One can even make a healthy sandwich from sourdough, wholegrain bread and a medley of vegetables, mushrooms and green leaves and some healthy cheeses.

Meals in a bowl can be inspired by a cross-section of Asian and South American dishes. Add avocados, when they are in season, to a bowl with wholegrain millets and a lentil and pumpkin curry. Or try a mix of stir-fried vegetables with tofu and unprocessed rice.

Let your culinary imagination run wild and you will approach lunch every day with joy and excitement. If you find yourself hungry in between lunch and dinner, put down that samosa or batata vada! Keep a box of dried fruit handy or perhaps eat a bowl of oatmeal with seeds around teatime. Smoothies also satiate hunger pangs, and help you get in some vital vegetables and fruit. Replace sugar with honey.

Burps are the stomach's red light. Stop eating much before you burp

You can eat your way to a century. The Okinawa islands in Japan have the highest number of people in the world over 100 years old. They eat mainly vegetables, whole grains and fish. But more importantly, they have a cultural practice called Hara Hachi Bu – to stop eating when you are about 80 per cent full. And this is the key factor to their longevity.

Having said that, it's hard to tell when we are 80 per cent full. How do we know for sure? Amazingly, our bodies do send us reports. And the most effective and communicative one is the burp. Burps are the red light of our stomachs, that clearly tell us that you're full, you have to stop sending down more food! Try to stop eating before you feel a burp surfacing.

Another way to limit food intake is through portion control, where you eat as much as you want, not as much as you think you want. You can do this by choosing a smaller plate. A large plate makes food appear less, versus a small plate that will look filled up and thus is psychologically more filling, satiating the hunger of our mind.

Keep it simple

At home we translate the simplicity of a small plate into simplicity of menu. In much of South India, including Mysore, Karnataka, where I live, meals consist majorly of rasam, sambar, rice and vegetables. We also eat a lot of salads like kosambari, which is made with split pulses, seasoned with mustard seeds. The legumes we use are usually bengal gram and green gram, which we mix with grated vegetables like beetroot, cucumber and carrot. We add generous amounts of root vegetables with sprouts and banana stem, which is high in fibre, to our salads. The one thing we don't do is complicate our food habits.

Our food is not fancy. It's simple, fresh and wholesome. Everywhere in South India you will find variations of the same balanced meal. Carbohydrates come in the form of red rice or ragi balls, protein from millets and dals, vitamins and minerals from vegetables and fruits, fats in the form of ghee. A simple South Indian meal is perfectly balanced and has everything the body needs.

Think about your food, but don't overthink it. If you are confused about how to start eating healthy, begin with what's always been cooked at home. Your staple food menu should be your first drawing board. Then, begin substituting the ingredients by choosing healthier options. Switch your cooking oil to a healthier one (look for cold-pressed, unprocessed, organic oils, especially those with a low smoking point), switch to red rice from white, go for organic vegetables rather than the usual fare. Once you've done this, you can experiment with other foods and cuisines too. Most people skip these steps because they think these improvements are tough to implement when you've always eaten a certain way.

Others may think such simple steps boring and want to jump straight to fancy and international ingredients which in the long run is hard to sustain. As the world becomes smaller, returning to these habits means we can move towards living more sustainable lives. High food demands all year round cause huge water stress and loss of biodiversity.[5] This also increases the risk of eating pesticide-laden or genetically modified foods, all of which lead to an increased toxicity in our bodies and the environment. The bottom line – don't complicate food; stick to tried-and-tested and clean eating traditions passed down from your ancestors.

Eat traditionally

About 400 years ago, the Portuguese arrived in Andhra Pradesh and brought with them tomatoes, which soon pushed out the traditionally used tamarind from its role as the sour ingredient added to legumes to make them more digestible.[6] Soon though, entire villages came down with fluorosis – a disease that causes permanent deformities – because the water in those areas had large amounts of naturally occurring fluoride. Research later determined that tamarind binds with fluoride to prevent it from entering the body.

We see a similar trend today. Due to rising incomes and access to international cultures, Indians are eating out more frequently. Today, we crave pizza, pasta, fries and burgers all the time.

Traditional foods and methods of cooking are being discarded in favour of Western diets rich in junk food. This is mostly because we've come to think that eating Western foods takes us up the social and economic ladder. But I've never heard anything as crazy as this.

When term begins in Mysore, I see many of my Western students eating dosas and idlis. But this doesn't agree with them in the long run. They suffer from cramps, indigestion and loose motions. How can a stomach that's not used to eating spices adapt to them in one season? I too can't eat foreign food. I will eat an occasional pizza because of my children, but it doesn't work for my body. I don't feel good. I can't even eat North Indian food. I don't mind the occasional roti, but in the afternoon I must have rice.

Cuisines across the world have developed differently because of a simple reason – availability of produce. And so our diet is strongly dependent on where we live, the climate and whether our ancestors ate foods rich in protein or fibre. While climate, terrain and availability of certain foods determines what finds its way on to your plate, there is also something called genetic memory. Carl Jung refers to it as the memory presented at birth through our DNA from our ancestors. It is what makes us who we are. How we look, behave, function, interact and react to our environment. Modernization has enabled us to ignore our genetic memory and this has taken us far from our ancestral diets, causing diabetes, obesity and cardiovascular diseases the world over. Journalist Michael Pollan writes that populations that eat a wide range of traditional foods generally don't suffer from chronic diseases. These diets run the gamut from those high in fat (the Inuit in Greenland who subsists largely on seal blubber) to ones high in carbohydrate (Central American Indians subsist largely on maize and beans) to others that are rich in protein (Masai tribesmen in Africa live chiefly on cattle blood, meat and milk).

Foods that come from your ancestors suit your body and help you live longer. Follow old traditions, don't throw out recipes handed down by your grandparents without a second thought. Our foods are different even from what our neighbour is eating.

If we stick to eating traditional foods, it will automatically mean we are eating seasonal produce. Mangoes in the summer and oranges in the winter. Gourds in the summer and carrot and cauliflower in the winter. Seasonal foods give us the most nutrients, simply because they are fresh. Do some research about the fruit and vegetables available in season, and then choose those when you are out shopping.

~

Since the time we have existed as thinking, sentient beings, from the ancient Greeks to our own epic heroes from the Mahabharata and the Ramayana, we have been enamoured by the idea of immortality. And is it really as complicated as our good old heroes from the epics made it out to be?

Honestly if I can do it, so can you. I have shown you the first and most important step in the journey towards good health, now let's turn our attention to how yogis eat and what sets them apart.

~

- Eat less to reverse ageing.
- Eat slowly.
- Explore traditional recipes to cure modern lifestyle diseases.
- Cook your own food to infuse it with love.
- Drink warm water to flush out toxins.

2

Eat Like a Yogi

You may be overwhelmed by the changes we spoke about in the previous chapter. But I am here to help you in your journey to discover an ageless you. The secret to a yogi's diet is simply a focus on what foods are healing, light, nutritious and filled with energy. We eat foods that keep our focus sharp and our minds clear.

In the pages that follow, I will share with you how my grandfather, my family and I have eaten for generations. With my wife's help, I have added some recipes to help you understand how we consume essential ingredients in healthy, traditional, wholesome preparations. Now we will look at what yogis eat.

What yogis eat

Here are the main foods that make up a yogi's diet. Some of these foods are also sacred because they are the building blocks of all energy and life for humans.

1. Yogis eat foods that grow above the ground

'Those who have incorrect food habits are unfit to undertake yoga,' said Krishnamacharya in *Yoga Makaranda*.

And so it is that yogis try to consume the right food in the right manner.

In Ayurveda, human beings have been described by three basic temperaments or gunas – tamas (darkness), rajas (activity), and sattva (purity). These gunas dictate the personality, behaviour and mental make-up one is likely to have.

These gunas can also be attributed to the food we eat. For example, sattvic foods are light, calming, filled with energy, and make us feel joyful when consumed. These foods are legumes, grains, fruit, climbing vegetables and sprouts.

Rajasic foods are usually stimulants and tempting things that bring to the fore emotions of aggression, ego, passion and control. For example, chocolate and coffee are well-known stimulants. However, on a side note, both coffee and chocolate contain polyphenols or antioxidants, and are good in small doses. Some rajasic foods are salmon, tuna, eggs, chicken, alcohol, tea, sugar.

Tamasic foods are usually overprocessed or fried, and include red meat and deli meats and are stimulants of laziness, desire for sex, greed and possessiveness. These foods are hard to digest.

Everyone has a mixture of all three gunas, with a predilection and excess of one or the other. Our diets should ideally have all three gunas in different portions depending on whether we need to be calm, active, energetic, creative or grounded. Rajasic and tamasic foods when eaten in excess make our minds violent or lazy depending on which guna is unbalanced. A rajasic diet with an excess of onion, garlic, coffee, teas and alcohol makes one restless, angry and passionate. A tamasic diet with meats, dairy, processed foods makes us dull and lethargic.

Yogis eat sattvic food because it keeps them sprightly, light on the feet, creative, fresh and filled with healthy thoughts. It helps in yoga practice and keeps their minds alert and active. It is a fundamental reason yogis enjoy good health.

An easy way to tell if a certain vegetable is sattvic or not is to see if it grows below or above the ground. Foods that grow above the soil are usually sattvic, while those that grow below the soil are most often rajasic.

Today, research coming out of universities and doctors has proven that vegetarians live longer. A study by the Transnational Health Science and Technology Institute in Faridabad found that the rural Indian's gut being more used to eating vegetarian foods is populated by gram positive anti-inflammatory bacteria – the good kind, versus the bad disease-causing kind, which are gram negative.

Another study states that vegetarians tend to consume less saturated fat and cholesterol. Vegetables are full of vitamins C and E (that ensure our heart is pumping well, our immune system is strong, our eyes are sharp and our lungs powerful), dietary fibres (that regulate our healthy morning ablutions and help us feel full for longer), folic acid (whose job is to create red blood cells), and potassium and magnesium are credited with improving brain health and fighting inflammation. We all know that phytochemicals come from colourful fruits and vegetables and contain flavonoids that are powerhouses of antioxidants and carotenoids, which make carrots so beneficial for the eyes. This is why a colourful variety of fruits and vegetables is recommended to prevent problems of the heart and even cancer.

One of the simplest food rules is from journalist Michael Pollan, boiled down as he says, to seven words: 'Eat food. Not too much. Mostly plants.'

2. Rice

Indians have been eating rice since 2000 BCE. We love our rice and eat it in beautiful white mounds on our plates. So much so that in our native languages, we often use the word 'rice' to mean a meal. Rice is a staple grain in our diet as it is a carbohydrate that provides us with energy for a day of physical work. Rice is also sweet and cooling. It cures pitta and stimulates vata. During times of illness we know it as the healing food – khichdi.

Traditionally menstruating women, children and the elderly are given the water rice is washed in to drink, as this boosts metabolism. Unprocessed rice – brown or red rice – with its hull on is the most nutritious, as processing removes important nutrients.

My grandma would also drink rice water. The starch of rice was made from cooking rice in a brass pot and then straining the water. To this salt was added, and then ghee, mustard seeds and coriander leaves. Of course, today we cook rice in a pressure cooker, so we lose the healthy rice water that is made from the traditional method. This very nutritious fluid gives energy, cures gut issues and prevents dehydration and diarrhoea.

Here's a great way to enjoy rice as my wife prepares it. This delicious and simple recipe adds zest to rice with lemon and crunchy chana dal.

Tangy lemon rice

Ingredients:
    1 cup cooked rice
    3 teaspoons groundnut oil
    ¼ teaspoon mustard seeds
    ¼ teaspoon chana dal
    ¼ teaspoon urad dal
    4 green chillies
    2 medium-sized onions
    ¼ cup curry leaves
    Coriander leaves to garnish
    Juice of 1 lemon
    Himalayan pink salt to taste

Method:
- Boil the rice and keep it aside.
- Next take a kadai/pan, add three spoons of oil. Let it heat, add mustard seeds, wait until they splutter.
- Add chana and urad dal and fry the dals until golden brown.
- Then add the chopped green chillies and onions and let the onions fry until they turn golden brown. Add salt and lemon juice.
- Lastly, add the cooked rice and mix it well. Garnish with coriander leaves and curry leaves. The lemon rice is ready to serve.

Tip: Replace the onions with green peas and capsicum to give the lemon rice a twist.

3. Milk

Both my grandfather and Krishnamacharya loved milk. They drank two glasses a day. I drink a glass of warm milk every day an hour before going to bed, with badam and kesar added to it for additional goodness and taste.

Milk is one of the ingredients of panchamrita – the five foods Hindus use in worship. Milk is sattvic. Along with rice, milk has long been another staple in Indian diets. Milk nourishes the tissues and helps balance your doshas. Milk is also a source of calcium for our bones.

Today, milk has a bad reputation in modern dietary conversation. Unfortunately, adulteration and pesticides have made it difficult to digest. Because nowadays milk is pasteurized, all the benefits of raw milk are effectively lost. According to Ayurveda, warm milk fresh from a cow is easiest to digest. But we may not all have access to that. Find organic, healthy sources for dairy in your diet, preferably from indigenous cows.

Milk is thick, heavy (unctuous) and slow to digest.

Milk also becomes easier to digest when heated with spices such as saffron, turmeric, black pepper and cinnamon as they reduce its mucus causing effects.

If you find the lactose in milk hard to digest (which is what happens when you lack the lactase enzyme required to break down lactose) try cottage cheese (where lactose is converted to the easier-to-digest lactic acid), yogurt or ghee (both of which are low in lactose) at home. Drink milk warm when you can as that helps you to digest it. Drink warm milk before going to bed to help you sleep better, but wait an hour or so after eating your food.

Here is a delicious dessert recipe made with milk that is perfect after a spicy meal.

Semiya payasam (vermicelli milk dessert) recipe

Ingredients:
   250 gm semiya roasted
   1½ litre milk
   3 tablespoons ghee
   10 cashews
   8 raisins
   ¾ spoon green cardamom powder
   225 gm sugar or jaggery

Method:
- In a pot, add milk and boil until the milk turns a little thick in consistency.
- Add semiyan to the milk and boil for about six to seven minutes, until the semiyan turns slightly soft.
- Add cardamom powder and sugar or jaggery and boil for a few minutes, just so that it mixes well.
- Heat the ghee in a small pan, add cashews and raisins and fry until cashew nuts turn golden brown. Keep the flame low. Then pour this mixture over the payasam, mix it well and serve hot.

4. Ghee

Prepared from clarified white butter, ghee is one of the five ingredients that make panchamrita. Ghee has now caught the imagination of the West and is popularly called magic ghee.

My grandfather used to say,

Ghrtena vardhate buddhih āyuh ksīrena vardhate |
Śākhena vardhate vyādhih māmsam māmsena vardhate ||

Ghee increases our intellect, milk increases our lifespan, vegetable increases our diseases – some vegetables, like potato, brinjal, tomato etc., flesh increases our fatness.

This means a spoon or two of ghee every day sharpens your mind, if you want a long life drink milk.

In South India, ghee is a common household ingredient. Even sambar, which is full of all kinds of beneficial ingredients like dals, vegetables, tamarind, turmeric and other spices, has one very essential ingredient, for taste and for health – ghee. Men in rural India who consumed large amounts of ghee were found to have a lower prevalence of coronary heart diseases. At home, we don't use oils as much as ghee.

Ghee lubricates the body and joints and is also a source of butyrate acid, a healthy, short chain fatty acid that is excellent for the health of the stomach wall, as it nourishes and reduces inflammation of the gut. It increases good bacteria in the gut and aids healthy elimination in the colon.

People who have excessive vata or those who are prone to both constipation and flatulence should introduce ghee into their daily diet.

It's extremely important to get your ghee from reliable sources or to make it at home. Commercially manufactured ghee runs the risk of adulteration which can cause heart problems. Pure ghee will never cause such problems.

Jois household tip:
For constipation, heat and drink about 20/30 ml of ghee at night. This allows and facilitates elimination.

5. Curd and pickles

Your gut is inhabited by a world of microbiomes in a carefully curated balance of good guys and bad guys. Very much like anything else in the world, this balance is important for your body to function healthily. Good bacteria protects you against the inflammation and infections caused when bad bacteria dominates, that can lead to a condition called gut dysbiosis.

Food poisoning, processed food and alcohol addiction or even an antibiotic course can deplete your gut of good bacteria. When gut flora becomes upset with an increase in bad bacteria, food begins to putrefy in the intestines and leads to digestive issues like bloating, constipation, candida, gastroesophageal reflux disease (GERD), acid reflux and gas or even skin and lung infections.

Strengthen your immune system with fermented foods. A healthy gut full of friendly bacteria from probiotic foods can handle everything from inflammation and allergies to autoimmune disorders.

Dahi is the star among Indian fermented foods. This lightweight, pitta-cooling food is a very important part of Indian diets. In K.T. Achaya's bible for food lovers, *Indian Food: A Historical Companion*, the author says Akbar started all his meals with curd and rice, which is an interesting take on our habits of ending meals with curd. At home, our family eats curd rice after each meal to cool the system, especially if a particularly spicy meal has disturbed our digestion.

Every Indian home has its own method for setting

a bowl of dahi. Go back to those customs of making dahi at home. Avoid buying packaged yogurt as it is not only sold in non-biodegradable materials like tetrapacks, but also has additives like sugar and preservatives.

For those who are lactose intolerant, lactose in milk becomes lactic acid during the fermentation of milk, making it easier to digest yogurt. Yogurt is also a good source of calcium.

A word of caution. Since dahi is heavy with kapha, it should be avoided at night, as the body undergoes an increase in kapha after sundown. Dahi should also be avoided in the winter as it is cooling and may not be digested easily in cold weather, causing it to putrefy inside one's body.

Dosas and idlis, made from fermented rice, are other probiotic rich staples in our diet.

Curd rice recipe

Ingredients:
    1 cup cooked rice
    1 cup fresh curd
    ½ cup milk
    Himalayan pink salt to taste
    2 green chillies

½ teaspoon mustard seeds
½ teaspoon cumin seeds
2 teaspoons ghee
¼ cup coriander leaves
½ cup pomegranate
½ cup green seedless grapes

Method:
- In a big bowl, add cooked rice, curd, milk, salt, coriander leaves, pomegranate, green grapes and mix well.
- Take a small pan, heat the ghee, add the mustard seeds, let the mustard seeds splutter, then add cumin seeds and green chillies.
- Fry for two minutes and pour over the curd rice and mix well and serve.

Other fermented foods like kimchi, sauerkraut and kombucha also help balance stomach pH, reducing the effects of low gastric juice secretion, commomly known as indigestion.

Pickles have a long history both in India and abroad. In 2030 BCE, pickled cucumbers were transported from the Himalayas to the Tigris Valley. Even Cleopatra attributed her good looks to a diet of pickles.

Pickling (with small amounts of Himalayan pink salt and oil) is an ancient Indian practice, known for being a rich source of probiotics. Home-made pickles are excellent because they help secrete digestive enzymes which start the process of digestion in the mouth. Pickled green mangoes or amlas are rich in vitamin C, and make for savoury sides to your meals.

While pickling, try to choose recipes that are brine (salt water) based, instead of oil based, and when using oil, choose cold-pressed oils over refined oils. One can even try swapping jaggery for refined sugar. Avoid oily or salty pickles if you are diabetic or suffer from hypertension. Those with excess of pitta should also avoid pickles, as pitta is a heating dosha.

Raw mango pickle

This recipe for raw mango pickle is special to the Jois family.

Ingredients:
    1 kg raw mango
    75 gm mustard seeds
    300 gm red chillies (200 gm crushed and
    100 gm whole)

2 teaspoons turmeric powder
Himalayan salt to taste
1 tablespoon asafoetida
Ceramic jar (traditional pickling jar)

For seasoning:
4 tablespoons oil (preferably organic, unrefined mustard oil)
½ teaspoon mustard seeds

Method:
- Wash the mangoes well as you will be using them whole with the skin. Cut the washed raw mangoes into small cubes. Transfer the mangoes into the pickle jar.
- For the masala, grind the red chillies, mustard seeds and turmeric together to make a powder.
- Now add salt to the mangoes and mix well.
- Then add the masala powder and asafoetida and mix well.
- Heat the oil and add the mustard seeds, and heat till they crackle.
- Cool and then add to pickle jar and mix well.
- Close the lid of the pickle jar and keep for three days.

6. Coconut

Used to bless new homes, broken to seal marriages, coconuts are considered sacred in India and used in many Hindu religious ceremonies. It's no wonder they find their way into so many of our meals in South India. In our home, coconut oil is used in all our cooking. Almost every single dish, from salads and vegetables to chutneys, is made from or garnished with coconut meat or milk. Even lentils are sometimes cooked in coconut oil.

Coconuts are a blessing because they are easily available to those of us living in a tropical area. They are full of natural saturated fats that increase good cholesterol. Coconuts are a medium-chain fatty acid that help boost metabolism and aid in fat loss. The meat of the coconut is packed with vitamin B and is a source of protein, so ensure you eat it after drinking the water.

Coconut water is an excellent beverage in the summer. Here in Mysore you will find a coconut vendor at every street corner. It's full of electrolytes and antioxidants and is very refreshing. Coconut water is also very good when you are sick, as it hydrates and detoxifies. But you shouldn't drink too much in the winter as it is high in vata, which can cause the build-up of phlegm and colds and coughs. People who suffer from asthma should also stay away from it or consume it in moderation.

Sprinkling grated coconut over your foods or making a coconut chutney with green chillies and mustard seeds is a staple across most cuisines in the South. Here's the recipe for a delicious coconut chutney that we make every day.

Coconut chutney recipe

Ingredients:
  1 cup freshly grated coconut
  4 green chillies
  ¼ cup roasted split chana dal or Bengal gram
  ¼ cup coriander leaves
  ¼ cup curry leaves
  1 teaspoon tamarind paste
  1 onion (optional)
  1 tablespoon oil
  ¼ tablespoon urad dal
  ¼ tablespoon mustard seeds
  Himalayan pink salt to taste

Method:
- In a pan, heat one tablespoon of oil.
- Add green chillies and fry for three minutes. Close the lid carefully, as the green chillies may splutter.
- Add freshly grated coconut and fry for five minutes.
- Cool the mixture and grind with tamarind paste, salt, coriander leaves, curry leaves, roasted spilt dals and a little water. Ensure this is ground to a coarse texture.
- In a pan, spoon in some oil, add mustard seeds and heat until they splutter.
- Then add the urad dal and fry until golden brown. Pour this over the chutney and mix well. Serve with dosa, idli or chapatti.

7. *Jaggery*

Legend has it that the first meal Gautama Buddha ate when he came out of his meditation was payasam made with jaggery. Jaggery is an excellent source of energy when taken in small doses, especially when we are weak and lacking in nutrition.

We were never denied sweets as children and would occasionally have an ice cream as a treat, but payasam was our most beloved sweat treat. This simple, delicious traditional dessert is made with vermicelli, dal or broken rice, with garnishes of coconut, cardamom, jaggery and poppy seeds. It is an excellent coolant in the summer. And you can get a little high from the poppy seeds if you eat too much! Don't forget poppy seeds are what opium is derived from.

In India we are blessed with a multitude of unprocessed sugars – the good kind – like jaggery or gur.

Diets high in refined and unnatural sugars, such as sodas, desserts, candy, white sugar and processed foods like breakfast cereals and ketchup are extremely harmful as they worsen your body's regulation of insulin, leading to obesity and heart disease.

Traditionally, we prepare many dishes in our home with jaggery, adding it even to sambar. I prefer taking the recommended dose of sugar in my diet (in 2014 WHO recommended not more than six teaspoons a day) in the form of fruit or jaggery. Jaggery is a complex sugar (versus refined white sugar) and takes longer to digest, thereby providing the body with energy for a longer time as opposed to white, processed sugar. Jaggery, an unprocessed derivative of cane sugar, is made without chemicals, versus white sugar, and so it contains more vitamins and minerals. Jaggery is also excellent for preventing chest congestions and coughs and colds. Add a little to your foods (see sambar recipe below from my wife Shruthi) or perhaps even eat a teaspoon of it after your meals as digestive.

Always remember that even jaggery and honey must be taken in moderation.

Carrot and green beans sambar

Ingredients:
  - ¼ kg carrots
  - ¼ kg green beans
  - 1 cup toor dal
  - ¼ cup chana dal
  - 5 pieces dry red chilli
  - 1 teaspoon poppy seeds
  - 1 teaspoon methi seeds
  - 1 stick cinnamon
  - ¾ cup coriander seeds
  - 1½ cup freshly grated coconut
  - 1 teaspoon grated jaggery
  - 2 teaspoons tamarind paste
  - 2 tablespoons ghee
  - ½ teaspoon mustard seeds
  - ½ teaspoon turmeric powder
  - Himalayan pink salt to taste

Method:

- Cut the carrots into small cubes and green beans into small pieces.
- In a pressure cooker wash the toor dal twice and then add carrot, beans, turmeric, one teaspoon ghee and two cups of water and cook.
- Wait until the second whistle, then switch off the flame and let the cooker cool.

For sambar powder:

- Heat a kadai. Add the chana dal, half a teaspoon of ghee and fry until the dal turns golden brown.
- Add the methi seeds with a little ghee and fry until golden brown. Then the add coriander seeds, fry that too.
- Add dry red chillies and fry in ghee until the chillies are crisp, and then add the poppy seeds. Poppy seeds fry fast and can burn, so be careful.
- Then fry the cinnamon stick in ghee for three minutes.
- Cool the mixture and grind with grated coconut to make a paste.
- Boil the cooked dal and vegetables for five minutes.
- Add the tamarind paste, salt and jaggery and boil again for five minutes.

- Then add the sambar powder paste and boil again for ten minutes.
- Finally heat one teaspoon of ghee.
- Add mustard seeds and let them splutter.
- Pour over the sambar, mix well and serve hot with rice.

8. Spices

In 1498 after ten whole months of adventure Vasco da Gama's men arrived at the port of Calicut. As his men got off their ship they yelled 'for Christ and spices!'

Though Vasco da Gama's request for a stalk of pepper infuriated the Calicut court, the potentate calmly responded, 'You can take our pepper, but you will never take our rains.' He knew pepper needed Kerala's strong monsoons and would never survive anywhere else.

Throughout history explorers travelled across many oceans at great risk for spices in India. And for good reason were pices considered more valuable than precious metals.

Spices do not just add mouth-watering flavours to our food. Across India you will find cuisines that explore the wonderful aspects of spices each with extraordinary properties that can heal a variety of illnesses.

The Upanishads state 'from earth sprang herbs, from herbs food, from food seed, from seed man'. Spices are the source of us as human beings. They balance out our doshas and alter the nature of foods to make them more digestible. Think for a minute of pepper. This hot and pungent spice decreases kapha and vata, counters pitta and is sprinkled on cold foods like cucumbers to counter their coldness. Similarly, milk is heated with turmeric to make it lighter and lentils always have a sprinkling of the magical spice turmeric to prevent them from making our blood impure.

Jois household tip:
I asked my wife for help in compiling a list of spice blends with specific medicinal properties. Here are some commonly found spices that will give your local chemist stiff competition.

1. *Allergies and coughs*: Trikatu – long pepper, ginger and pepper – makes a wonderful medicine that is used to treat coughs, colds and fevers.
2. *Constipation*: Spices improve digestion so much that one can see why they are used before meals (pink salt and ginger), while cooking (asafoetida and nutmeg) and after (fennel). Triphala made with amalaki, bibhitaki and haritaki helps to internally cleanse your system by aiding

bowel movements. Nutmeg, another spice used generously in our kitchens, is medicinally used in times of indigestion. When added to foods it can improve cognitive function. Use this zesty spice in desserts, cakes or tea as a supplement for sugar.

3. *Daily detox*: Ginger is 'the universal remedy' and balances and controls all three doshas. A mixture of fresh ginger juice, lemon juice, black pepper and turmeric added to warm water and had every morning can help restore digestive juices and cleanse your system of toxins. Keep extracted ginger juice in your refrigerator; this amazing SOS heals a host of problems. Ginger juice fights headaches, nausea and even normalizes cholesterol. Add a teaspoon to your juices, teas or morning cup of turmeric and lemon warm water, or take half a teaspoon with honey at night.

4. *Antioxidant tea*: Cardamom is a diuretic and promotes heart and lung health. It helps promote the passage of food through the intestines, and cures indigestion and gas. Clove is an anti-inflammatory and cinnamon, anti-microbial. Add a few pods of cardamom, a few peppercorns, a stick of cinnamon, a few slices of ginger to water and boil. Add honey for taste. Don't boil honey. You can even have cardamom as is, if feeling nauseous.

5. *Injuries*: Apply turmeric and ghee to scrapes and cuts. Or simply sprinkle powdered turmeric and watch your scrape, scratch or even punctured skin heal immediately. Just remember to clean all injuries thoroughly before applying any medicine.

6. *Fatigue*: Another powerful healing root is sarsaparilla, that can help everything from fatigue, indigestion to liver and immunity disorders that show on the skin like psoriasis and eczema. It is also excellent against migraines. Add a small pinch to soda or milk, or find it as homoeopathy drops or Ayurvedic tablets. Please consult an Ayurvedic doctor before taking these as medicine.

7. *Acid reflux*: Boil water with fenugreek, mint, cumin and fennel for an SOS cure against acid reflux or soak overnight and drink in the morning for a general healing of the digestive system. Fenugreek also helps diabetics control their blood sugar levels.

Yogis don't eat onions and garlic

Both my grandfather and his brother (a priest) were very spiritual men who never ate garlic or onions. Ancient Hindu tradition dictates that Brahmins avoid spices like onions and garlic as they contain rajasic and tamasic properties that excite the mind and slow down your path to enlightenment.

Personally, I have never liked garlic in my food, as I find its flavour too strong and its powerful smell affects my practice. When you chant you need to concentrate, and your pronunciation is very important, and at certain times your tongue can twist if you eat garlic.

Sanskrit texts have called garlic 'The Disgusting' or Rahu's Residue, as it sprang from Rahu's blood when he was beheaded. It is an elixir for the body, but can also increase tamas in the mind, making a person intolerant and overstimulated.

On the contrary Ayurveda loves garlic and onions for its potential to kill harmful bacteria and reduce cholesterol. So, eat both onion and garlic in small portions or use them for medicinal purposes only. Onions cooked with your food, or consumed in juice form or raw, stimulate the heart, promote bile production and reduce blood sugar.

Jois household tip:
- To cure an earache or infection crush two pods of garlic in a little bit of mustard oil and heat. Once cooled pour this oil inside your ear. This analgesic helps fight infection.
- A mixture of honey and ginger juice, about one teaspoon, can cure fevers and colds.

Sharath's power protein drink

I drink a powerful protein drink that is great for vegetarians. I always recommend this to my vegetarian students, who have high protein requirements because of their strenuous Ashtanga practice. You also get iron from the copper vessel and lots of strength from the dal.

Ingredients:

A handful of moong dal

1 cup water

1 teaspoon jaggery

A copper vessel, bowl or glass

Time: Overnight. Prepare this before you sleep.

Method:

- Clean the moong dal by washing it a few times until the water is no longer white. Soak the dal in fresh water in a copper vessel, cover it and keep overnight.

- In the morning, put the moong dal, water, and jaggery in a blender to make a smoothie-like drink.

Is meat bad for us?

This is the most commonly asked question by my international students: Is eating meat bad?

I was born into a Brahmin family, and so I have never eaten meat in my life. Dals and milk compensate for the lack of animal protein in my diet. But my answer often surprises people.

Yes, of course, meat is bad for people who are committed yogis because (1) it goes against the fundamental principle of ahimsa and I am strongly opposed to killing and eating another life that has memories, feelings and emotions; (2) it is a rajasic food that causes restlessness and also lethargy; (3) factory farming today means that most meat is loaded with harmful chemicals and antibiotics; and (4) it is hard to digest versus vegetables.

Imagine this – a big vegetarian thali takes five to six hours to leave the body. Red meats can take up to a day. People who eat a lot of meat often find they get constipated because of its high iron content, which leads to problems in their GI tract and digestive organs, as meats take longer to leave your body. Other health risks from diets high in meat are type 2 diabetes, coronary heart disease, stroke and even a higher probability of certain cancers.

But eating meat isn't always a bad thing. There are many reasons that people choose a carnivorous diet. Perhaps you have a geographical necessity to eat meat or your doctor has advised you to eat it for health reasons, or if you have been brought up on a non-vegetarian diet. For people who find it tough to give up meat, try and eat it in moderate quantities. Meat is not bad for you, but those who choose to eat it should find the most responsible, non-toxic ways to consume it.

If you eat meats, be mindful of what you buy. Look for meats that are ethically farmed, antibiotic-free and pasture raised. Even if this choice is more expensive. And if you must eat meat, do so in the afternoon because it is easier to digest at that time of the day.

How yogis eat

Eating is not just about food. How we eat also matters. In your new journey as a fire worshipper, you must review how you eat. Do you eat watching TV? Or in front of your desktop? Do you eat alone or with people? Yogis have mastered the art of eating correctly, that's why we rarely suffer from indigestion.

It is very important to listen to your body. You should not ignore signs like heaviness or indigestion after certain foods. You must learn to slow down. Sit down and eat. Perhaps even sit cross-legged. Breathe in between bites. Eat slowly, chewing your food to savour all the flavours. Turn off all screens to try to focus simply on eating, while eating. Here are a few ways to change the way you eat so you can get the best from every bite.

Yogis always eat home-cooked meals

Yogis live by the old Vedic saying *svayam pāka*, which means one should always cook one's own food. That is the only way you can control what you're eating and how much oil, salt and spices you use. It also ensures hygiene standards. But cooking your own food also means that you can infuse your food with love, cook with care, feel reverence and love for your foods.

When I was growing up, my grandmother or my mother would cook for the family. Of course, times have changed, and now we have a cook who helps us cook for our children. When I travel, I still cook for myself

Cooking at home is the best thing you can do for yourself. Indians have always cooked most of their meals at home. Visiting a hotel or a restaurant was an occasional treat. And dinner at home with the family was a daily, important social activity. Back then, we mostly lived in joint families where one or two of the women would dedicate themselves to cooking. Things have changed drastically. In urban India, about 60 per cent young people eat out at least thrice a month, while Indians eat out without their family about 75 per cent of the time. Young middle-class millennials spend roughly 10 per cent of their total food expenditure on dining out and purchasing cooked meals from restaurants, caterers and canteens. Unfortunately, our desire to eat out and post beautiful images of our food on social media has made us forget how to cook, what to cook and what real nutrition is. We also end up buying a lot of partially cooked foods from supermarkets that require little preparation, but these foods are made and stored using preservatives and made with substandard salts and spices. Eating out or ordering in, especially eating fast food, has made us perhaps the only country that is grappling with both obesity and malnutrition at the same time, as equally serious problems. Isn't that a sad irony?

According to the World Food Program, the rates of obesity and diabetes in India increased between 2010 and 2014, and 9.5 per cent of Indian adults are diagnosed with diabetes, while 4.9 per cent suffer from obesity.

Preparing your meals in advance

On a weekend, plan your menu for the coming week. Write it down and stick it on your fridge. Then go out and get what you need.

Prepare curries and dals for the week. Freeze and store in clear stackable storage boxes in the fridge. Even vegetables can be chopped and stored in airtight containers, so that they can be used over a few meals. However, don't keep cut vegetables for more than a day as they lose their nutrients once they are cut. Keep ready to make mixes of oatmeal and dried fruits in your fridge, so you can easily cook those in the morning. Similarly, make salad mixes of vegetables a few days in advance, with a side dressing that you can mix on the spot.

This is how you can move from eating a fast food sandwich or burger, on the go, to actually eating foods you have thoughtfully put together the previous night.

Today, as more women join the workforce, things have changed. I'm all for women going out and working. But it's sad that most men have not yet learned to be self-sufficient in the kitchen. It is important that cooking doesn't fall solely on the shoulders of the woman. If both partners know how to cook, then they can avoid eating out.

Many of my foreign students cook their own meals to take to work and I encourage working people to also find solutions to this. With a little meal planning you can cook on Sunday or the weekend, for the whole week. Explore quick, easy-to-make recipes of wholesome meals with fresh, locally bought produce.

Yogis eat at the same time every day

Even though my meals follow the unusual schedule of my teaching routine, I make sure that I eat at the same time every day. After my own practice, the first thing I eat is a small bowl of oatmeal, sprinkled with a mix of spices such as cinnamon and cardamom and a sprinkling of seeds. This is at about 3.30 a.m. Then I go to teach. At 9 a.m., I have a small salad along with my protein shake or a smoothie or juice.

Around 11.30 a.m. I have a big meal. I started eating lunch earlier after my bout of acid reflux. In the evening, between 4.30 p.m. and 5 p.m. I have a chapatti with a little vegetable and dal, and then a glass of spiced milk before sleeping.

The point I'm making is that you should eat at the same time every day because our bodies like habits. And practice makes habit. Science is catching up with this today. A study found that people who ate at random times suffered from high blood pressure and saw an increase in body mass index (BMI), versus people who had strict eating schedules.[1]

On the other hand Ayurveda has long recognized the importance of regulating food intake according to the circadian rhythm. Our bodies regulate our doshas according to the clock. In the mornings, from 6 a.m. till 10 a.m. kapha increases. Waking up before 6 a.m. in a peaceful time, when vata dominates, makes you energised for the day. When vata dominates you can be very productive, so eat a light meal at 6 a.m. once you have exercised and meditated, and use the midday sun to finish tasks and achieve goals.

In the afternoon till 2 p.m. pitta is dominant. Your biggest meal should be now, when the natural world is warm and your digestive fire or jathra agni is awake. It is easy for the body to digest heavy meals during these hours.

And from then until 6 p.m. is for vata. Governed by ether and space, vata is generous to creativity, so ideate and solve problems during this time of the day.

The best time for dinner is between 7 and 7.30 p.m. Make this a light meal, as your body is seeing an increase in kapha again and is starting to slow down. Drink hot tea or warm milk at this time to help your body wind down.

At night, your pitta increases between 10 p.m. and 2 a.m. This is when your body detoxes, and when you should stop eating. But if you have a long working day, eat your dinner at 9.30 p.m. but ensure you have a two-hour gap before you go to sleep.

The gaps between your meals depend ultimately on you and your body issues. Please consult a doctor before making any drastic changes in your food schedule. But stick to the timing you have set.

After any exercise remember to wait at least half an hour to forty minutes before you eat. All your organs are twisted and turned after exercising or practising yoga. You must allow your body to settle down internally.

Yogis always drink warm water

At home, we always serve water warm. It is common to find restaurants in South India also doing the same. Wherever I travel, I take my flask of hot water with me. And there is a specific reason for this. Warm water aids digestion, whereas cold water constricts our muscles and extinguishes our digestive fire. Bacteria thrives in cold water. When you heat water, bacteria dies. Warm water improves blood circulation, helps alleviate headaches, and even halts premature ageing, by ridding the body of toxins. This almost diuretic early morning flush helps cleanse the body while repairing skin cells and increasing elasticity.[2]

In the morning when you wake up, before your morning ablutions, drink two to three glasses of warm water to flush out toxins accumulated from the previous day.

In your third glass of water, squeeze in some lime juice. Lime is full of polyphenol, a micronutrient that has been known to help with diseases like cholesterol and blood pressure. Even though lemon is acidic, once it's inside you, it becomes alkaline. Lemon water is the key to keeping your pH levels balanced and your body alkaline.

You can also do a lukewarm salt water gargle to cleanse your mouth. This heals any soreness you may have, removes bacteria and helps you speak clearly without any impediments of smell or pain.

After a meal wait forty minutes to an hour to drink water. This is so your food and water don't mix, and prevent the dilution of essential digestive juices.

If you can, store water in a copper container at night and cover it. Drink this water first thing in the morning. The water absorbs copper from the vessel. This copper-rich water is antimicrobial, antioxidant and anti-inflammatory and balances out all three doshas.

Yogis eat with their hands

According to the Vedas, each finger represents the five elements – earth, water, fire, ether and air – that are stimulated in the foods when we eat. Your fingers have nerve endings that convey texture and temperature of the food you are touching to your brain, adding another notch to the sensory activity. Eating should be a pleasurable activity.

Indian cuisine has foods that are only meant to be eaten with our hands. Even though eating habits have changed drastically today, I can't imagine eating rasam and rice, rotis and dal and dosas and chutney with cutlery.

Eating with your hands is also cleaner as we wash our hands before consuming our food. You also tend to eat consciously and slowly, versus eating with cutlery.

Be mindful, slow down and feel the difference in your food when you eat with your hands.

Yogis always walk after a meal

Our former president Dr A.P.J. Abdul Kalam is a good example of yogic living. He was known to walk for an hour after his meals, even in the sweltering heat of Delhi. He was also a vegetarian.

Walking after a meal is an extremely good practice that helps digest meals better. This activity[3] speeds up the rate at which food moves through your body. Even a twenty-minute walk can lower post-meal blood sugar levels.[4]

Do not go to bed immediately after eating. And you can achieve this by not eating late at night. If leaving the house at night isn't easy, find an activity to do that doesn't allow you to sit. Wash the dishes, tidy your house, play with your kids. I'm sure you'll find something to do.

~

- Eat foods that grow above the ground, otherwise known as sattvic foods.
- Don't throw out rice water – as it's full of important nutrients.
- Boil milk with turmeric, saffron and black pepper to make it easier to digest.
- Add ghee to your food regularly as this lubricates joints and helps us live a longer, pain-free life.
- Pre-prepare foods to avoid reaching for unhealthy foods during the week.
- Drink water warm to improve blood circulation and digestion.

3

How to Perfect Your Daily Routine

The great Hatha Yoga teacher Sri Ramamohana Brahmachari asked T. Krishnamacharya for a simple payment in exchange for his teachings. He told him to return to his home, begin teaching, and start a family.

Contrary to the idea of yogis being brahmacharis, or bachelors, T. Krishnamacharya and Guruji were both householder yogis. This is a legacy I continue to carry forward today. Like my grandfather, I have chosen to be connected with society, to have human interactions and to have a family. Yoga has many different practices that are passed down from guru to shishya. Mine came from two great teachers. And it works beautifully for me, making everyone around me happy and positive.

We are not in an age where yogis go into the forests to seek enlightenment. But if we were, it would've been much easier for me to be a yogi. Yes, I wouldn't have the comforts of modern life, but I would have had all the time to live, study and practise to be a yogi. There would be no disturbances in my sadhana.

Householder yogis have a more difficult time, because we must balance our spiritual, physical and intellectual sadhana and the innate desire to be a sanyasi that comes with that sadhana, with the responsibilities of looking after our families. Over the last few decades I have learned how to balance these aspects of my life – my sadhana, my practice, my students and my family. I think life is really all about management. Each day has twenty-four hours. We spend eight of those sleeping. Of the remaining sixteen hours, we need to be careful how we manage our time. And this is where a householder yogi like myself can show you how to make the best of those hours we have.

A yogi lives a productive life because he or she appreciates and understands the importance of living in the present. We know that every moment wasted will never return, and so we make the best use of our time, by living by the rules of nature. We can see the entrapments of modernity that bind and limit people, and most of all we can see how people go astray by disregarding some simple habits that can be incorporated into their daily routine.

In this chapter, I am going to talk about what a healthy and meaningful routine should be like. These are simple, tradition-based guidelines. But, trust me, even those of us familiar with these practices aren't following them the correct way.

We cannot achieve longevity or a peaceful life by eating ostentatious meals and buying expensive gadgets. In fact, it's the opposite.

Don't worry, I won't tell you to throw away your phone just yet! Instead we will look at what you can do differently from the time your alarm clock rings to when you go to bed at night. Together, we can explore how your daily routine can be perfected so that you get the best out of it.

The untapped potential of the sacred hour

Let's start with when your day begins. No one takes the adage, 'early to bed, early to rise', more seriously than yogis. When I am not teaching I wake up to practise around 3 a.m. When I am teaching I wake up at 1 a.m. to practise and start teaching by 3.30 a.m. This is perhaps one of the many reasons people think yogis are crazy. But this is not a time chosen at random to torment us. This is what the Vedas call the Brahma Muhurta – an hour and a half before sunrise. This is considered the most sacred time of the day.

Translated literally to the Creator Hour (Brahma being the creator and Muhurta being time), this is the time of stillness, peace, purity and creativity. The hours of the creator. If you are seeking stillness of the mind or even a good idea that eludes you, try waking up at this hour to think and reflect on your problems. At this time, your mind and energies are calm and you may find that answers come much easier than when the world is awake. When everything is still, people are still asleep and the air is pure, your mind and energies are at peace. Early mornings are important because you can control the rest of the day from here.

In Ashtanga Hridayam, this hour is described as '*brahmi muhurtam uttishthet swastho rakshartham ayusha: tatra sarvartha shantyartham smareccha madhusudanam*'. This can be roughly translated to waking up during the Brahma Muhurat gives us perfect health and helps us live a long life.

Brahma Muharat is one of the greatest potentials that we overlook and haven't unlocked. This is the hour that holds the secrets to happiness and success, but only if we are willing to put in the hard work. We know no good thing comes for free, and yogis through the times are familiar with the power and price of waking up early.

Of course, we yogis do crazy things, and I don't expect this will suit your lifestyle. What I urge you to do is try it out once a week to start with. Wake up at 3.30 a.m. and watch what happens to your mind and how your day progresses. At first, you may find yourself completely exhausted and drained by 8 a.m.! But persistence is the key. And if you're seeking a long and peaceful life, what are a few early mornings, right?

The potency of prayer

In Vedanta philosophy there is a much-loved story of a man who mistakes a rope for a snake in the night and goes to arduous lengths to avoid it. The next day by daylight he sees it for what it is and realizes how darkness can lead to fears and superstitions.

I think of prayer as a stabilizing and grounding experience that leads us away from fear and darkness. A request to God to guide us into light. In the Gayatri Mantra, the chant 'Om Bhur Bhuva Swaha' is our prayer to be delivered from ignorance.

The idea of prayer can be controversial especially when ascribed to a particular religion. But I always tell my students that you do not have to be religious to pray. Religion is personal. Who you pray to is not of anyone's concern. Each one of us has our own istadevata or cherished god.

Most Indian families have a prayer, very personal to them, that they recite daily, or more often than not, in desperate times. Perhaps you have one too. Haven't you ever found yourself calling out to a higher power in times of need?

Prayers are the yoga of the mind. They help calm us, cast light on our troubles and bring about a sense of hope in times of trouble. Focused prayer or chanting is about centring the mind. Time and again, studies have proven that prayer or a daily meditation improves relaxation, enhances focus and concentration and lowers blood pressure.[1] In a study Christian nuns in prayer and Tibetan monks in meditation were found to have increased dopamine levels – the hormone which makes us happy.[2] This is simply one amongst a multitude of studies that have found regular prayer boosts the immune system, deactivates genes that trigger inflammation and cell death and helps increase longevity.[3]

Reciting a chant – or a japa as it's called in Sanskrit – is proven to be mentally and emotionally reinvigorating. Chanting creates auditory vibrations that help you evolve spiritually and help you connect with the Supreme Being. But most importantly, chanting helps us connect with ourselves

So how can we make prayer a part of our lives?

Find a chant that sits well on your tongue. It could be anything – a family chant, your own personal chant, repeating the word Om, or even the words of a poem that inspires you. At certain times of the day, remove yourself from a hectic work or home environment to chant. Once you have established a habit, try and find time to chant first thing in the morning and the last thing before you go to bed.

Early mornings are best for prayer because they can refresh your mind and bring positive energies the whole day. Before you sleep, do japa every night for as long as you can. This will help you unwind from a long day of work, so that you can go to sleep easily and wake up the next morning unencumbered from the day before.

A twenty-four-hour cycle doesn't comprise only one emotion. We can be joyous, sad, anxious, jealous, irritable and scared from hour to hour. So many of our emotions are yesterday's leftovers. When emotions from the previous day aren't dealt with and cleansed, they coagulate and build up in our mind, making it tough to clear them later. Yoga isn't just a physical practice; it's a mental and emotional endeavour too. Banishing negativity from your mind is part of that mental practice. There is a simple rule that sums up most of our lives. Your thoughts will dictate the outcome of your life. More precisely, you think therefore you are. When your thoughts are negative, your actions will be the same. A nightly japa helps rid us of the emotions that have passed through us from morning to evening of the current day. It is a closure to the day gone by.

For those who prefer meditating, concentrate on something – an object, or a spot of light in the distance. Or try sitting in silence and letting your thoughts come and go, slowly working to silence your brain.

Saucha, inside and out

Prayer gives us the strength to clear our mind of negativity. Taking that concept forward are these teachings from the Bhagavad Gita – purity of body comes from cleanliness of body, purity of mind comes from truthfulness and non-violence, and purity of thought comes from reflection, silence and peace of mind.[4] Here, let us discuss purity of the body.

First amongst Patanjali's niyamas is saucha, or cleanliness. This is a very important limb of Ashtanga. Saucha literally means cleanliness, purity and clearness. There are two kinds of saucha, external or baher saucha – which involves keeping your body, clothes and environment clean.

If you can keep your surroundings both inside your home and outside your home clean, then your mind will also be clean. Each one of us plays an important role in keeping our country clean, and we should never forget or underestimate that.

Antar saucha means to keep your body clean from the inside. For this, you must exercise to get rid of toxins and keep your nervous system pure and you must practise positive thinking. Over a period of time, correct breathing techniques and a regular asana practice can help you develop positive and affirmative thoughts.

Yoga is prayer. It's much more than exercise. So, all yogis bathe before their yoga practice. We come to our mats clean and pure. It is similar to how we wash our hands and feet in waterbodies outside a place of worship.

We meet all kinds of people during the course of a typical day. These simple social encounters lead to a lot of toxins being deposited on you through conversation and touch. Bathing in the morning and at night helps us get rid of these accumulated toxins and unwanted energies. When you are physically and mentally fresh, you will have a different experience of your asana practice and your day ahead.

Having said that, don't bathe too often or use too much soap. I see so many people who are addicted to sanitizers. Harsh alcohol-based sanitizers leach your skin of its natural bacteria and kill your immunity. Bathe twice a day – once in the morning and after you come back from work. Use soap sparingly, if only once a day, or opt for natural cleansing products like soap nut or shikakai (a natural soaping agent).

Walk barefoot to earth yourself

When was the last time you just lay on the grass and watched the sky and the clouds float by? When was the last time you felt the ground beneath your feet?

It saddens me how disconnected we are from the earth today. Most of us never feel the earth like we once used to. But how can we do so when we live in fifteen-story buildings, move around in cars and airplanes? We can't. But don't lose hope.

In a study, Chicago's Rush Medical College found that the impact on people's knees was lowered by 12 per cent when they walked barefoot. The study says we walk better without the impediment of large thick rubber soles. Our feet have 200,000 nerve endings. Shoes ruin the natural curvature of the feet, they cover these nerve endings, almost suffocating them.

I like to imagine our bodies as divided according to the five elements, from your feet to your knees is earth. From your thighs along your hips you're water. Your stomach is jathra agni or fire and your lungs are air. And everything neck upwards is ether. Ayurveda also has specific mud and herb therapies for people, where they are buried knee-deep in treated mud. These treatments stimulate pressure points in our feet that our nervous system is connected to, thus exercising and activating them. This is very similar to how acupuncture and acupressure work, where energy moves when certain points in the body are stimulated.

One way to keep our legs and feet connected and strong is by walking barefoot. At home, I always walk barefoot. It helps me connect with the earth. This practice, known as earthing, is spiritually healing and can also cure physical problems. Earthing has helped decrease blood glucose in diabetics and regulate endocrine[5] and nervous system functions. Better still, twenty minutes of barefoot walking on mud or grass can make your energies flow uninterrupted and stimulate your legs and feet, ease inflammation and insomnia, and even beat depression.

While I prefer nature over those materials used to construct our floors, I understand it's not always easy to access them. But don't give up. Just walking barefoot in your home can be a small but productive exercise.

Sleep in a dark room

When I sleep I ensure no light comes into my room from outside. Neither from the moon, nor from artificial lights on the streets.

This is very essential for your body to create melatonin when you sleep. Produced in the pineal gland, melatonin is what makes us sleepy at night. The natural production of melatonin has been hampered by the advent of electricity and digital screens, which in turn has created in us a host of problems from anxiety to insomnia.

It's important to create a dark environment to sleep in, with blackout curtains if necessary and even an eye mask. Red night lights are useful for children's rooms or if you need some light to make your way to the bathroom at night.

Sleep enough, but not too much

Chimpanzees choose the bed that will give them the best sleep. Bats sleep upside down. An albatross is known to be able to sleep whilst flying, and sharks can sleep while they swim. Humans are the only creatures for whom familiarity and routine make for the best sleep.

People come to me when they have trouble sleeping. Insomnia, the inability to sleep, is on the rise today because people have too many anxious thoughts running in their minds. Problems with work top the list.

Lack of sleep can be dangerous because it is known to cause cardiovascular diseases, compromised immune function, diabetes and stress. Sleep is what charges our bodies, and without it we will descend into madness.

So, how can we go to sleep without tossing and turning all night long?

The first is to be physically tired. Include physical activity in your life to induce this. The other, less often mentioned factor, is habit. Sleep, like every other physiological aspect in our life, is heavily dependent on habit. If we've trained ourselves to go to bed at 9.30 p.m. every night, we'll gradually find that by 9.30 p.m. we can barely keep our eyes open. You should try and adopt a fixed routine. If possible, go to bed as early as you can and wake up early. Fix a time for yourself and stick to it as strictly as you can.

On an average, try to be in bed by 9.30 p.m. and wake up between 5.30 and 6 a.m. Eight hours is the maximum you should sleep. Do not get less than six hours of sleep. On the other hand, if you sleep more than eight hours, you will become lethargic and lazy. Sleeping too much during the day increases kapha.

I have often fought this battle to sleep enough. And anyone who has as gruelling a schedule as mine will understand this. However, since I have habituated my body for those months of the year when I am teaching, to sleep for fewer hours at night, even when I am not teaching I can't sleep more than five hours. I wake up early every single day of the year no matter what my plans for the day are. But I have ensured I get my prescribed hours of sleep in the afternoon. Even for those of you who work night shifts or keep irregular work hours, like I do, it's very important to get your mandatory seven to eight hours of sleep whenever you can in the day. Therefore, power naps are crucial for people like us.[6]

Power naps are wonderful to restore alertness and to help you de-stress, whether you are shuffling between boardrooms or are a new mother with an infant on an irregular schedule.[7] In fact, they are more effective than coffee, with benefits that are less varied and longer lasting. Short naps, of not more than fifteen to twenty minutes, at that moment when your energy dips in the day, between 1 p.m. and 3 p.m., are excellent to renew learning, reduce stress and improve your mood. Just lie down or rest your head on the desk and close your eyes for fifteen minutes. If you can't sleep, close your eyes and rest. Or simply sit silently for ten to fifteen minutes. Especially when you have been working for five to six hours, this can be very relaxing. It's a reboot for your brain.

Never sleep with your head to the north, as the earth's magnetic field reduces your peripheral blood flow and this drains your energy and your positive thoughts. It can even increase irritation, restlessness and confusion. Sleeping towards the west can cause violent dreams. Sleep to the east for meditative sleep, or to the south for deep, physically restful sleep.

Disconnect one day of the week (perhaps on Sunday)

When I say disconnect, I mean both online and offline.

I would love to tell you all to toss all your gadgets out of the window, and focus on whatever is in front of you in real life, but I do recognize the crux of this problem. We are all addicted to our gadgets. They are more than just playthings; they facilitate our work and keep us connected to those we love. But I worry about the time we spend on them and how they affect our lives.

Gadgets may have made our lives extremely comfortable, and we can't even imagine life without them, but I think they've also made us very unhealthy, both physically and emotionally. Depression is at its highest in human history. And it's no surprise that the biggest culprit of our global misery is social media.

What happens when an acquaintance posts something positive about their life, whether it's a new job, a vacation, a new haircut or a new baby on social media? What do you feel? Happiness? Envy? Guilt about feeling envious? Do you feel like you could do better?

Of course, we'd like to feel happy for them, but we

are only human. But so many times we also experience that fleeting sense of jealousy, anxiety, sadness or desire. We secretly hanker for what other people have. We can't help this fundamental human characteristic. The grass is, unfortunately, always greener on the other side.

And that's why social media companies are billion-dollar companies. Because they know this. They know that human beings can be insecure, seek appreciation, and can desire endlessly. So they keep us hooked. In small doses, social media is good for us, it helps us connect and helps with our work. But it also causes anxiety by making us feel bad about ourselves, it fosters an environment of ruthless competition and mindless imitation. It also makes us uninterested in the world around us, and lazy and physically inactive. If you feel this pressure and anxiety every time you look into your phone and want a change of scene, try something radical . . . switch off your devices over a weekend. I know! that sounds crazy. But connect with the people right in front of you. Take a break from the anxiety they cause. You don't even realize how much until you feel that panic rising when you can't find your phone. If that's not anxiety, I don't know what is.

To have a balanced life, we must be judicious about how we use our gadgets. Our gadgets lead us into an attractive cyber world, but remember, it's all maya. An illusion. See how you cut out stress by taking a break from your phone just once a week.

A study in 2016 found 46 per cent of the workforce in organizations in India suffers from some kind of stress or the other, 43 per cent have a skewed BMI of which 30 per cent are at diabetic risk, 30 per cent have hypertension. In another report, Indian millennials put in the most number of hours a week at fifty-two hours. These scary statistics prove the abysmal lack of work–life balance in the workforce today. While offices can also introduce more progressive policies, on an individual level we must not just give up all control to our employers. One of the ways in which we can regain control is by rediscovering an ability to disconnect. Try to do this at the end of each work-day, or on weekends.

Spend your Sunday with family or by yourself. Perhaps you can use this time to think about the other aspects of life, perhaps poetry and philosophy, indulge in a hobby, get in some RnR or just simply unwind in a park.

Socializing excessively makes us worry unnecessarily and makes life complex. In life we must build strong barriers and know when to cut off from people. Don't be unnecessarily involved in people's stories. Yes, you should care for those around you, but you cannot take on all their worries. You will be no help to them or to yourself if you cannot help yourself.

~

- Wake up early to have control over your day.
- Walk barefoot to stimulate and heal your body.
- Sleep eight hours to heal and charge your body.
- Reinvigorate yourself with prayer.
- Disconnect from the internet to find happiness.

4

Fast Once Every Fifteen Days and Other Secrets to Cleanse Your Body

'There is no acquisition superior to that of righteousness, and no penance superior to fasting,' Bhishma advised Yudhishthira on his deathbed. 'It was by fasts that the deities have succeeded in becoming denizens of heaven. Viswamitra passed a thousand celestial years, confining himself every day to only one meal, and as a consequence thereof attained to the status of Brahmana. Chyavana and Jamadagni and Vasishtha and Gautama and Bhrigu – all these great rishis endued with the virtue of forgiveness, have attained to heaven through observance of fasts.'

This passage from Book 13 of the Mahabharata highlights the importance of fasting, an act that has always been closely linked to immortality and divinity in most religions. It is a powerful tool that has been used both politically and spiritually from time immemorial. Fasting is a practice common across religions. Hindus fast according to the lunar calendar, during Navratra or on days of the week reserved for particular deities. On Ramazan when Muslims fast, they don't just abstain from food and drink, they also focus on purifying their souls through good behaviour. Across the year, Jews fast on six different days as repentance, out of which Yom Kippur is the most holy. Christians of most churches observe Lent, while Buddhist monks and nuns fast during times of intense meditation and don't eat anything after noon as a regular practice. Mormons are encouraged to fast on the first Sunday of every month.

Throughout India's history from Mahatma Gandhi to Irom Sharmila, activists have fasted for their politics. Gandhi may have had an unimpressive initiation into the world of fasting, as he records in his book, *My Experiments with Truth*, 'Having been born in a Vaishnava family and of a mother who was given to keeping all sorts of hard vows, I had observed, while in India, the Ekadashi and other fasts, but in doing so I had merely copied my mother and sought to please my parents.' Yet, later his decision to fast unto death for the freedom of India was so powerful it changed the history of this country. In his book *Non-Violent Resistance* (*Satyagraha*), Gandhi says that while spiritual fasting is tapas, 'fasting is a potent weapon in the satyagraha armoury. It cannot be taken by everyone. Mere physical capacity to take it is no qualification for it. It is of no use without a living faith in God. It should never be a mechanical effort or a mere limitation. It must come from the depth of one's soul. It is, therefore, always rare.'

So why do people fast?

While political leaders like Gandhi did it to drive home a point, others do it as penance, humility, cleansing, a path to a higher spiritual order, and a way to remind themselves of the value and importance of food which we usually take for granted.

Whatever the reason, we cannot take lightly the innumerable benefits of fasting and cleansing. In this chapter I am going to take you through the many ways we can cleanse and purge our bodies of the many toxins we take in on a daily basis.

Today toxins are ubiquitous in our lives. They are everywhere: air pollution inside and outside, processed foods, chemicals, plastic and garbage, the list is endless. However, we can look to the ancient practices of yoga and Ayurveda to remove these toxins.

Purification is an integral part of yogic practice. Traditional cleanses like shat kriyas and pranayama are prescribed to clear the blockages and tension hindering us in our everyday life, but they are also very effective in fighting a host of allergies that often lead to other severe and chronic health issues. Outside of the shat kriyas, your cleansing can start anywhere – cleave plastic from your life as much as possible, cut down on addictions such as tea and coffee, start an asana practice and adopt practices such as fasting or shat kriyas.

Read on to understand how you can cleanse your life of toxins.

Fast – give your stomach a day off

My grandfather and Krishnamacharya fasted on the eleventh day after moon day, on Ekadashi. On that day they would only drink beverages, mostly just milk. I have adopted a similar fasting routine.

Reset your system with regular fasts. The first positive impact is on the digestive system. It gives your stomach a break from its constant job of having to digest food. Like any other machine, your digestive system needs rest. But the benefits of fasting aren't just limited to your digestive tract. A one-day fast gives your organs a break from working hard to accumulate digestive juices and helps your body get rid of toxins and build immunity.

Science has shown that fasting reverses ageing and builds immunity. Studies amongst people who fast regularly have shown improvements in blood pressure, cholesterol and insulin sensitivity. Fasting has also been seen to retard the growth of tumours and augment chemotherapy by sensitizing a range of cancer cell types to chemotherapy.

Simply by fasting once a week or once a month your entire system can get an overhaul.

Yogis believe that the food we eat over the course of thirty-two days gets transformed into a single drop of blood. After thirty-two drops of blood, thirty-two days must pass for these drops to become one drop of vitality or immortality. After thirty-two drops of vitality have been generated, and again, thirty-two days have passed, one drop of amrita bindu or the nectar of immortality is produced and stored in the head.

Amrita bindu is stored in the pineal gland. Think of it as ambrosia, the nectar of the gods. The flow of amrita bindu through you can be thought of as the moon flooding one's body. Amrita bindu is what makes the body resistant to toxins. It lends strength and shine to body and mind. When the store of bindu decreases one's lifespan is shortened. A healthy bindu preserves health and mental clarity.

The bindu is preserved by inversions such as Viparita Karani, where you lie down with your legs up a wall, or Sirsasana or Sarvangasana for those who have a regular practice and are familiar with it. When you fast, your digestive juices rest and so does the amrita bindu.

If you've never fasted before, start with once a fortnight. Juice or vegetable fasts are easy introductory fasts. Once you are comfortable going a whole day without solid foods, see if you can do it twice a month.

Fasting is an extreme measure. Pay attention to your body when you are doing it. If you are diabetic or prone to acid reflux, fasting may not suit you. If you have high levels of acidity and need to eat small light meals, then try and eat a small, healthy snack every few hours. If you are pre-diabetic (when your blood sugar levels are higher than normal) or have mild hypertension you can start by skipping a meal. But ensure you consult your doctor before adopting any of these dietary changes. If you are over forty years old and have never fasted before, your body may find it difficult to adapt to new eating habits. So it is vital to be careful when adopting fasting practices.

Kriyas to purge your body of toxins

The popular purification methods written about in great detail in the *Hatha Yoga Pradipika* are shat kriyas. These ancient yogic techniques were used by rishis to ensure that their bodies were clean and healthy for spiritual practices. So what are shat kriyas?

Shat karmas or shat kriyas (literally translated to six methods) are prescribed to cleanse internal organs as detailed by Swami Swatmarama in the fifteenth and sixteenth centuries. By unblocking areas of tension, shat kriyas as tools can help us remove poisons and toxins from our bodies. The six kriyas are neti (which includes jala and sutra), dhauti, basti, nauli, kapalbhati and trataka. Each of these are to be done under proper guidance. It is important that you learn how to do these kriyas from someone trained as a yoga guru. Avoid doing these kriyas on your own or through YouTube tutorials.

1. **Neti:** This practice clears the nasal passage and sinuses and stimulates a purging of toxins from the lymph system (the network of tissues and organs

that rid the body of toxins by carrying lymph, the infection-fighting fluid that contains white blood cells). Both jala and sutra neti are excellent cures for allergies, colds, bronchitis and asthma.

Sutra neti: Take a string of cotton and a rubber catheter and insert this through your right nostril. The thread will follow the rubber catheter in through your nasal cavity down into your throat and can be brought out from your mouth. Pull the thread back and forth thrice. Change sides to do it on the left side. This method needs practice and you may initially even see a little bit of blood as blood vessels can get damaged from the thread, but do not worry, as you will get comfortable with this method. You could even try to soak the thread in beeswax, like they would in the old days, to soften the thread.

Never do this without the requisite focus and mindfulness. If pain occurs, slow down, you may have been pulling too fast.

This kriya removes congestions and alleviates breathing problems that flare up in the winter or during allergy seasons. This is also very useful for people who often find that one nostril is more blocked than the other.

The best time for any kriya is early morning on an empty stomach. Avoid doing any kriya every day. Just two or three times a week is good enough.

Jala neti: This nasal irrigation technique is typically performed with a neti pot and is excellent for people who suffer from seasonal allergies. Using the side of the pot with the spout, pour lukewarm, distilled water mixed with a pinch of sea salt or Himalayan salt through one nostril. The water will automatically flow out through the other nostril, cleansing your nasal passage and removing dirt and mucus filled with bacteria. Breathe through your mouth.

People who have asthma should avoid jala neti unless they can do it under close supervision of a yoga teacher. Jala neti is not advised in cold weather as it can worsen a cold, and lead to phlegm build-up if water gets left behind in the nostril. Therefore, I recommend sutra neti even if it seems more difficult to master, as there is no fear of worsening congestion from this method.

2. **Dhauti:** Dhauti means purification. Instruction in this kriya includes methods to cleanse the tongue and eyes, ears, etc. Dhauti kriya includes different methods of cleansing the oesophagus and stomach, either by drinking large quantities of saline water, or by inserting a long thread down the throat. Practitioners who are familiar with dhauti kriya, having been guided by experts, will see allergies, acidity and even asthma cured with regular practise of this method.

    You must remember to be careful when doing these kriyas, as you can develop problems like anorexia and bulimia.

    Drink two litres of warm water with a teaspoon of salt in it. Drink quickly, standing upright. Bend forward, press your hand into your abdomen and extend the fingers of your other hand down the throat, to induce nausea, until all the water comes out. Perform on an empty stomach.

    Bhasti: This is a method for cleaning the bowels. Like an enema, water is drawn in from the anus to clean the colon. Another version involves the practitioner drinking many litres of saline water and flushing it out through the rectum to cleanse the intestine. This flushing happens through a series of twisting exercises that stimulate the intestine to purify the blood and detoxify the body. This helps with allergies and even skin diseases.

Nauli: This is the practice of contracting and rotating abdomen muscles to cure digestive disorders, by stimulating the jathra agni.

Trataka: This wonderful tool is used to remove mental toxicity. (Please refer to the chapter on meditation.) This helps age-related deterioration of the eyes. These exercises give your eye muscles flexibility.

Kapalbhati: This powerful breathing method helps dispel toxins from the deepest parts of the lungs and is done with other pranayama after asana practice. If you are new to yoga, I recommend pranayama (see next section) as a gentler and safer method to cleanse your body.

I strictly do not endorse the use of nauli, bhasti and dhauti methods, unless you are a seasoned practitioner and have an excellent teacher under whose guidance you can follow these cleanses. However, newcomers to yoga can practise neti, perhaps by seeking out a teacher who can show them the ropes.

Excessive shat kriyas are contraindicated if you have a sustained asana practice, because the practice already requires a lot of breathing. One must remember that shat kriyas only give temporary relief and should be used to complement your asana practice.

Oil baths release physical tension

Now that we have discussed all the different ways in which you can detoxify yourself internally, let's talk about the body's exterior. In Ashtanga Yoga, Saturday is the day off from practice. On this day, all yogis are advised to take an oil bath. An oil bath is different from a massage as in the former you simply apply the oil and massage for a few minutes into your skin and then sit with the oil on you allowing it to soak into your skin and muscles, versus a more physically intense, longer massage.

The heat created from the oil lubricates your joints and helps with pains, muscular discomfort and inflammations. This is a very powerful practice. Take it easy the day you have an oil bath, and avoid overstressing your body.

Oil baths taken once a week are excellent for aches and pains, and all kinds of inflammation and skin allergies. If you don't have access to an Ayurvedic centre that specializes in oil massages, you can do it yourself. The practice of self-massage is called abhyanga.

Use either coconut, castor or almond oil to do this. Castor oil is very thick. So, heat it to thin it down. Apply the oil to your head, wait fifteen minutes and then massage it on to the rest of your body. Make sure that when you rub, the oil on your body heats up with your palms. Then, wait for about ten to fifteen minutes. Use a mixture of shikakai (a natural soaping agent), soap-nut powder and arappu powder (made from the leaves of the *Albizia amara* tree) and hot water to wash the oil off your body. Work the powdered mix in a circular motion to remove the oil. A hot shower will further help you sweat the toxins out.

Avoid using an excess of powders, lotions and creams as these block your pores and don't let toxins leave your body.

Oil baths are so effective that I always advise my students not to get massages. I believe deep tissue massages damage the nervous system. Massages are good for people who don't do much exercise, but for those who are active and exercise every day, they don't

Castor oil as a purge for constipation

When I was a child, once every six months my grandfather would mix castor oil in my coffee to help my digestion. I used to run away from this noxious drink.

But castor oil is a wonderful laxative for those suffering from chronic constipation. As a child I was made to drink 35 to 50 ml of castor oil and then sit out in the sun. The oil was meant to heat up inside me and the toxins would be flushed out as we sweated and even the next day through a full diuretic purge.

Instead of this method you can add one tablespoon of castor oil to ginger tea a few nights in a row before sleeping, to help you cleanse your colon in the morning.

If you live in a cold country, try and find sonamukhi leaves (*Cassia angustifolia*). Boil the leaves and have a small cup of this digestive cleansing tea which stimulates a secretion of enzymes from the liver, making it an excellent laxative.

These are both very powerful purgatives, so it is important to use them carefully and be hydrated during the entire process.

need someone stomping on them, breaking their back and pushing them around.

If you lead a sedentary life, massages can get your blood circulating and bring movement to the body. Of course, a massage will never have the same benefits as regular exercise.

The one-cuppa rule

For years I used to say 'no coffee, no prana' to students who found it challenging to wake up early and come for asana practice, at a time when the rest of the world was sleeping. So they would ask me how I stayed awake, and alert, and I would say, 'Drink coffee!'

I started drinking coffee when I was around twelve years old. In South India, we have a long history of drinking coffee from medieval times. If you drink coffee in small amounts, it's good for you. But like anything else becoming addicted to it mitigates its effects. If you drink coffee through the day or are drinking it to lessen your anxiety and stress, then put that mug of coffee down, because it is doing you more harm than good. Coffee addiction can be a gateway to addiction to alcohol, food etc.

Asana – the ultimate detox

Sitting in a sauna or getting a massage is a good way to detox and unwind, but it doesn't hold a candle to physical exercise or an asana practice. Sweating helps eliminate toxins like BPA[1] (from plastic) and phthalates[2] (used in everything from cosmetics to paints) that enter our bodies from the things we use every day without a second thought. Regular exercise helps you burn fat and stops you from becoming an obesity statistic.

Yoga is the best form of exercise versus anything you choose to do in a gym. During yoga practice, one inhales and exhales deeply and consciously. This exercises your organs, allows the blood to circulate, thus eliminating toxins from your body, almost pushing or flushing them out of your body. Of course one also sweats while standing outdoors in the sun, but that is an external heat. An asana practice cleanses you internally.

When you inhale and exhale you activate your jathra agni or stomach fire. This is the prime agni that nourishes the other agnis. My grandfather used this analogy in *Yoga Mala*, but I will repeat it for those who may not have had the opportunity to read it. He says that gold comes from impurities. It is made by heating them up, in a process called smelting. Thus, impure particles born with the gold are separated from the precious metal.

Just like gold emerges from impurities when heated, when we exercise our blood gets heated – I like to think of it almost as being liquidized with easy movements. A combination of breathing techniques, exercise and yoga, makes our blood thin, warm, and ensures it flows unobstructed to all our organs, thereby nourishing the body. A disciplined yoga practice generates heat and energy inside us and in turn makes our blood circulate through the body. This means food is digested easily and digestive juices increase and toxins are efficiently eliminated.

On the other hand, if you have a regular asana and breathing practice you won't need panchakarma cleanses, unless you have serious digestion and health problems. Panchakarma is a detox that involves five (pancha) types of treatments to cleanse the body of toxins. Oil and steam therapies, lymphatic massages and enemas are amongst the treatments done to balance out the doshas and rid the body of accumulated toxins. But you can't do these and then get back to an unhealthy life. Panchakarma, like shat kiryas are not permanent cures; they only give us temporary relief. Yoga is the best permanent method to live a clean and toxin-free life.

Read on to find out more about incorporating asanas into your life to uncover the ultimate secret to agelessness.

~

- Fasting gives your digestion an overhaul.
- Fight allergies with the practise of shat kriyas.
- Take oil baths to release muscular tension in the body.
- Avoid massages as they damage the nervous system in the long run.

5

Ten Asanas are All You
Need to Do

Now that we have touched upon food, routine and habits, it is but obvious a yogi's book must talk about asana practice – the physical part of yoga. Perhaps you had a class somewhere once, or a family yoga teacher, or maybe you saw your first yoga lesson on television, and so you associate yoga with doing a series of bendy moves on a mat. However, you may be surprised to know that Patanjali in the Yoga Sutras gives no specific instructions about asana practice. Ancient rishis used asana to make their bodies strong and supple so that it could withstand rigorous meditation. Today, the physical aspect of yoga has become more important than the spiritual, because we find it easier to commit to a physical routine that to commit to a philosophy or a way of life. But the fascinating part of yoga is that even those who take the route of asana first will find themselves slowly but automatically coming around to the spiritual part of the practice, to explore and live their lives in a yogic manner both on and off the mat.

So why is asana practice important? Well, the most obvious reason is your health. The most common problems people come to me with are breathing and respiratory issues. One of the leading causes of death, air pollution kills seven million[1] people a year in urban areas across the world. And about 28 per cent of those deaths happen in India.[2]

Asanas not only strengthen your body against illnesses, they also cure illnesses that attack the body. You've read my story; it was the power of asana that healed my ailing childhood body.

Please remember to consult a doctor before beginning any exercise routine, especially if using it to heal a medical condition. This is not a replacement for medicine, but a powerful supplement when done properly.

Who is it good for?

Hathasya prathamāngatvāt āsanan pūrvamucyate |
Kuryāt tadāsanam sthairyam ārogyam ca angalāghavam ||[3]

Asanas are in first place as they form the first stage of Hatha Yoga. Asanas that make one firm, free from diseases, and light of limb.

Both the practice of yoga and a yoga practitioner can seem tough and intimidating. But anyone can do yoga. In this section I have included asanas that can be done by people who have never done a class in their life, or perhaps have done a few classes. There are asanas for people across all age groups. Please read all precautions and modifications carefully.

Vinyasa

Asana is nothing without a proper breathing technique. In Ashtanga, there is a special focus on breathing, as each asana is accompanied by strong inhalation and exhalation. We call this vinyasa – a breathing and movement system that has one breath for each movement. For example, in Surya Namaskara A, described later in this section, there are nine

Vinyasas. Asanas are organized in a way so you don't just learn a physical movement, but you also learn to inhale and exhale at the right time.

Vinyasas create internal heat that cleanses and strengthens your organs. And sweat, an important by-product of vinyasa, leaves your body along with diseases. With a focus on your respiratory organs through inhalation and exhalation, asana helps prepare your lungs for the next limb, which is pranayama.

A good method to remember when to breathe in and out – asanas with upward movements are governed by inhalations and those with downward movements with exhalations. When you reach up with your arms or your chest through your neck you inhale, and when you curl in or reach down you exhale.

The Ashtanga sequence

Ashtanga Yoga consists of six sets of sequences. Practitioners start with the Primary Series, after which some move on to the Intermediate Series. Very few of these will move on to the Advanced postures broken into four series, called Advanced A to D. The Primary Series, also called Yoga Chikitsa, literally means yoga therapy, and is required to make us healthy, get rid of disease and purify our bodies, through asanas and breathing techniques.

An Ashtanga sequence starts with the foundation sequence of Surya Namaskara A and B that helps warm up your body.

This is followed by standing postures like Trikonasana, Trikonasana B and Parshvakonasana. These work on an external level as they strengthen your legs, target fat and reduce your waist and stomach. At an internal level they work on your digestive and respiratory organs, both of which are strengthened with these standing postures.

One of the main purposes of your practice is to reduce your waist so that it is narrower than your upper body or chest, so as to avoid diseases like obesity. The *Hatha Yoga Pradipika* says,

Vapuḥ kṛśatvam vadane prasannatā
nādasphutatvam nayane sunirmale
arogatā bindujayo'gni dīpanam
nādī viśuddhir hathayoga laksanam

The signs of perfection in Hatha Yoga are: the body becomes lean, the speech eloquent, the inner sounds are distinctly heard, the eyes are clear and bright, the body is freed from all diseases, the seminal fluid is concentrated, the digestive fire is increased and the nadis are purified.

Simply put, when you have a thinner waist and lower abdomen you will automatically be healthy.

One then moves into forward bends. Asanas such as Baddha Konasana and Upavistha Konasana and Janu Sirsasana help lengthen your spine and the muscles along your upper body, legs and arms. They also help improve your breathing. An asana practice is what brings mental and physical stability to our bodies and our minds, so we can focus better on meditation or pranayama, be calm, strong and healthy and unlock the secrets of agelessness. Didn't I tell you there's no magic here.

Points to bear in mind before starting your asana practice

Time: Patience is key to a good asana practice. Yoga is unlike any other form of exercise. Asanas take time to perfect. It takes time to build up strength. There are no shortcuts. Start with a shorter practice and then keep adding asanas, as you get comfortable, stronger and more flexible.

Only when you practice every day will your muscles loosen up; your hips will rotate better, and your joints will open up. And as you get stronger, keep extending your practice time.

Start with a half-hour or forty-minute practice every day. Even this will show you a marked difference in your well-being. Your body will be better aligned, and your breath will become stronger, and you will find freedom and mobility in your body.

Benefits: Each asana has its own specific benefits that contribute to our overall health because it works on every single organ inside our body. For example, Baddha Konasana works on your digestive organs, while Urdhva Dhanurasana helps respiratory organs. Standing postures like Trikonasana, Utkatasana and Virabhadrasana work on your lower abdomen, while strengthening your legs. And in all these asanas, when you breathe consciously, your respiratory organs are also getting exercised. Pranayama is very beneficial for your respiratory organs.

A dedicated practice will make your body strong and healthy and rid you of recurring diseases. A strong asana practice also mitigates age-related injuries and strengthens your ability to heal, which becomes difficult as you get older. Asanas are extremely beneficial for people who battle anxiety, stress or have sleeping difficulties.

I cannot stress enough on the mental exercise one gets during an asana practice. Observe how when you are angry or sad your breathing becomes shallow and fractured and your heart rate increases or the act of yelling at someone or reacting angrily in traffic increases your heart rate. After your practice, the immediate benefit you will feel is peace of mind. Never skip Shavasana at the end.

Building flexibility and strength: Some people are blessed with stability, but no flexibility, or vice versa. To balance those two sides out, you need daily practice. Do not attempt too many asanas at once. Build up stamina, strength and flexibility by developing your asana practice day by day, and then slowly keep adding asanas. You will get there if you do these every day.

Sitting on the floor: Patanjali describes asana as sitting. To be sitting in a posture that is firm, yet relaxed. You must sit on the floor every day, so that your body gets used to it. Only then will you develop a certain flexibility.

Breathing: Initially during certain asanas, you will feel your breath is shallow and short, but this routine, practised regularly, will help regulate your breath, making each exhalation and inhale longer.

While doing your asanas, concentrate and breathe consciously. Breathing like this expands your upper body and increases your lung capacity. Ujjai breathing makes your breath powerful and strong.

Proper inhalation and exhalation calms us and reduces anger, emotional instability and distractions, all of which exist because of the lack of oxygen in our bodies.

Equipment: The best part about yoga is that all you need is comfortable clothes, a mat or rug and a little open space, and of course a willingness to heal your body, in order to live a long, healthy life.

Your daily asana practice sequence

1. Surya Namaskara A and B

Surya is the source of energy. It is life giving. Everything on earth is because of Surya. In Indian philosophy, Surya or the Sun is like the health minister, it is where you get all your vitamins and minerals from.

Ārogyam bhāskarāt icchet, that is, if you wish to get good health, you have to pray to the Sun God.[4]

When you do Surya Namaskara it is as if you are directing solar energy inside you, to your organs, to make your body healthy.

In yogic practice, we always start with Surya Namaskara: a prayer to Surya for its bounty. There are two parts of Surya Namaskara (A and B). The physical benefits of the two sequences of Surya Namaskara are manifold. Your body becomes warm and energetic with the movements, and your strength and stamina improve. Your entire body and all your organs are exercised by practising this set of postures.

Āditya hrdayam punyam sarvaśatru vināśanam |
Jayāvaham japennityam aksayyam paramam śivam ||

[This] holy [hymn] to the presiding deity of the sun,
if chanted fervently, will result in the destruction
of all [your] enemies and bring you victory and
unending supreme felicity.

Remember to perform the Surya Namaskara with proper concentration on alignment and your inhalations and exhalations.

To start with, do ten to fifteen sets of Surya Namaskara A and then five to eight repetitions of Surya Namaskara B. If you do this every day, you don't have to do any other exercise, as this is considered equal to a two-hour walk. Remember to end sitting in Padmasana with some slow breathing.

Surya Namaskara A

Method:

- Stand in Samasthitih (mountain pose) at attention. Hands by your side, knees together. Stand as if a thread is holding you up – running along your spine through the crown of your head. Inhale and exhale.

- Inhale and take both arms up, palms touching. Exhale and come down into Uttanasana A bending from the waist. Bring your head down last. Touch your forehead to your knees, if your hands don't reach the floor catch your shins. You can bend your knees depending on how tight your hamstrings are.

- Exhale and look up into Uttanasana B, place your hands on the floor and jump or step back and lower into a low plank or Chaturanga Dandasana. In a low plank keep your palms on the ground, elbows close to your chest. Ensure your shoulders are rotated out, and not collapsing into your chest. Keep your neck and back straight in one line. Keep your hips off the ground, but not too high that they

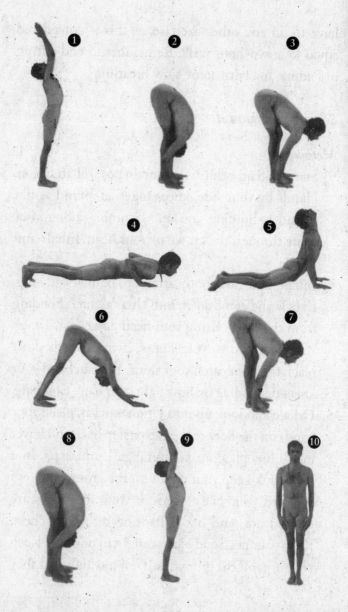

are outside the line made by your back and legs. Keep legs strong.

- Inhale and look up, coming into Urdhva Mukha Svanasana. Turn your toes out, so you're pressing into the tops of your feet. Stretch your back and neck long, pressing the hands. Stay off your knees if possible, keeping all weight on top of your feet. If you find this tough, keep your knees on the ground.

- Exhale, come into Adho Mukha Svanasana. Breathe here for five slow yogic breaths. Ensure your shoulders are rotated out. Practise this as if shrugging your shoulders away from your ears. Keep your neck in one line with your spine, and don't push your neck too much. Keep every point on the bottom of your feet connected to the ground, as much as possible. If your heels don't touch the ground initially, work slowly at the posture and you will see how your hamstrings open up to allow for full contact with the floor.

- Exhale your previous breath, inhale and jump or step forward and look up in Uttanasana B. Exhale and bend your head to your knees in Uttanasana A.

- Inhale with arms up, palms together. And exhale as you bring your arms down by your side back to Samasthitih.

Surya Namaskara B

Method:

- Stand in Samasthitih (mountain pose). This is an attention position. Hands by your side, knees together. Stand as if a thread is holding you up – running along your spine through the crown of your head. Inhale and exhale.

- Inhale, bring your arms up above your head, and bend your knees as if sitting in a chair, to go into Utkatasana.

- Exhale into Uttanasana A, head to your knees, or shins. Bend knees if hamstrings are tight.

- Inhale look up, keeping your hands where they are, and jump back from Uttanasana B into Chaturanga Dandasana. In a low plank keep your palms on the ground, elbows close to your chest. Ensure your shoulders are rotated out, don't collapse into your chest. Keep your neck and back straight in one line. Keep your hips off the ground, but not too high that are outside the line made by your back and legs. Keep legs strong.

- Inhale and look up, coming into Urdhva Mukha Svanasana. Turn your toes out, so you're pressing into the top of your feet. Stretch your back and neck long, pressing through the hands. Stay off your knees

Ten Asanas are All You Need to Do

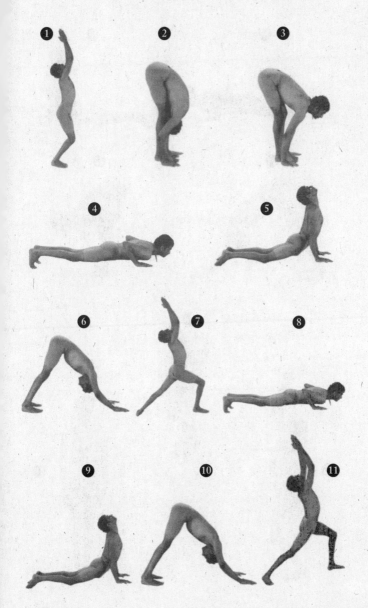

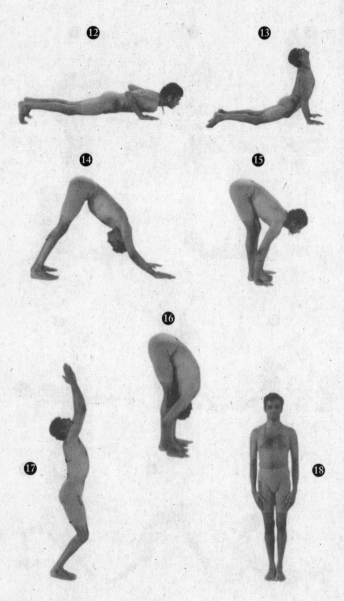

if possible, keeping all weight on top of your feet. If you find this tough, keep your knees on the ground. Exhale, come into Adho Mukha Svanasana.

- Inhale and step your right leg back into Virabhadrasana A. Bend your left knee, keeping your thigh parallel to the floor. Look up at your hands if you can, or straight in front of you.
- Exhale down into Chaturanga Dandasana, inhale up into Urdhva Mukha Svanasana and exhale back to Adho Mukha Svanasana.
- Inhale and step your left leg back into Virabhadrasana A. Bend your right knee parallel to the floor. Look up at your hands if you can, or straight in front of you.
- Exhale down into Chaturanga Dandasana, inhale up into Urdhva Mukha Svanasana and exhale back to Adho Mukha Svanasana. Breathe here for five slow yogic breaths. Ensure your shoulders are rotated out. Practice this as if shrugging your shoulders away from your ears. Keep your neck in one line to your spine, and don't push your neck too much. Keep feet on the ground as much as possible. If your heels don't touch the ground initially, work slowly at the posture and you will see how your hamstrings open up to allow for full contact with the floor.

- Exhale your last breath, inhale and jump or step forward and look up in Uttanasana B. Exhale, head to your knees in Uttanasana A.
- Inhale, bend your knees into Utkatasana.
- Exhale to Samasthitih.

After doing the Surya Namaskara sequences, you can practise the ten asanas I have explained below for a robust workout. These also provide a cure for a number of health issues.

2. Utthita Trikonasana A and B

In Sanskrit, utthita means extended and trikon means triangle. This asana is part of the Ashtanga standing sequence, and strengthens your legs while reducing fat from the sides of your waist. The perfect Utthita Trikonasana is to catch your big toes, but if you have a weak or tight back just catch your ankles or shins, until you are comfortable and find the flexibility to go deeper.

Note: If you have back problems, avoid twisting too much in Utthita Trikonasana. Pregnant women should avoid this asana. And people with lower back pain should also avoid it or not push themselves too much in this posture.

Utthita Trikonasana A

Method:

- Stand in Samasthitih.
- Inhale, jump or step to the right with legs spread three feet apart.
- Spread arms out to the side.
- Exhale, turn both feet to the right. Your left foot is turned slightly inwards. Bending from the waist go down sideways to catch your right big toe with your right thumb and forefinger and middle finger, or rest your hand on your shins if you can't reach your toe. Keep your chest facing forward, don't collapse into your leg in an effort to reach your toe. Lift your left arm straight up with your fingers pointed to the ceiling.

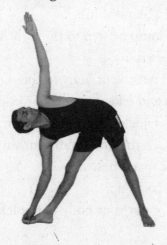

- Breathe five times.
- Inhale, come up.
- Exhale, turn the feet to the left, bending from the waist go down sideways, to catch your left big toe, with your left thumb and forefinger and middle finger. Rest your hand on your shins if you can't reach your toe. Keep your chest facing forward, don't collapse into your leg in an effort to reach your toe. Lift your right arm straight up with your fingers pointed to the ceiling.
- Breathe five times.
- Inhale, come up.

Utthita Trikonasana B

Method:
- Stand in Samasthitih.
- Inhale, jump or step to the right with legs spread three feet apart.
- Exhale, twist your body to the right, lift your left arm up and take it over the side, placing your left hand outside of the right foot, on the floor. If you can't reach the floor grab your shin, ankle or calf.
- Breathe five times.
- Inhale, come up.
- Exhale, twist your body to the left, lift your right

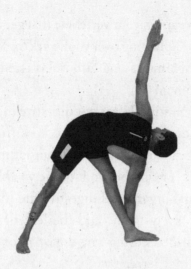

arm up and take it over the side, placing your right hand outside of the left foot, on the floor. If you can't reach the floor grab your shin, ankle or calf.
- Breathe five times.
- Inhale, come up.

3. *Pachimattasana*

Back pain is a ubiquitous part of our lives today, most of the time caused by bad lifestyle habits and routines. How we sit, work, sleep and stand creates all kinds of tension in our shoulders and back. This asana realigns our spine that could otherwise get compressed from sitting for long periods of time. It stretches the spine,

121

and creates gaps in your vertebrae that get compressed by sitting or hunching over your work for long periods of time. Pachimattasana also helps strengthen your lower abdomen.

This asana stimulates your digestive organs, where digestive juices or jathra agni comes from. As you inhale and exhale, you activate your Jathra Agni and just as if air is being blown into fire you blow air into your internal organs and digestive fire to increase it. This burns away toxins and the lower part of your body is purified curing any digestive or respiratory issues you may have.

When pregnant women practise Pachimattasana they should spread their legs and then do the forward bend, otherwise this will put pressure on the foetus.

Note: The counter pose to this is Purvattasana. This back-bend also helps with respiratory problems. The two asanas together are very important as they also purify your nervous system, and provide relief to people who suffer from tonsillitis.

Pachimattasana A

Method:
- Start in Dandasana. Dandasana is the foundation for all seating postures. Dand means stick, and in

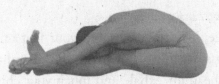

Pachimattasana A

this you are as straight as a stick both going up and down from the waist. Sit with your hips on the floor and your hands on either side of your hips, palms open and pressing into the floor, legs stretched out, big toes and heels touching. Press down from your heels, tighten the muscles of your legs and reach up from your spine, while rotating your shoulders back. Your chest neither puffs out, nor collapses.

- Inhale, reach forward from the waist and catch your big toes with your forefinger, middle finger and thumb, and lift your head up. Keep your back straight and don't bend at the neck. If you have difficulty catching your feet, hold your shins instead.
- Exhale, touch the head or chin to the knees and breathe five times.
- Inhale, head up. Exhale, release.

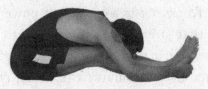

Pachimattasana variation

123

Pachimattasana variation

- Inhale, lock hands around your feet or hold the outer sides of your feet with both hands.
- Lift head up, exhale and touch your chin to your knees. Breathe five times.

Purvattasana

Method:

- Start in Dandasana.
- Inhale and exhale, take the hands back and one foot behind your hips with your fingertips facing your hips.
- Inhale, lift the hips up without hardening the buttocks and press your shoulder blades against each other to support the chest. Breathe five times.
- Your feet are on the ground, with your toes and heels touching. Try to keep the soles of your feet connected with the ground.
- Exhale and come down.

4. Baddha Konasana

Baddha Konasana is a basic, but powerful seated posture that strengthens the back, stretches and relieves tension in your hips and inner thighs. Baddha Konasana also stimulates the heart, circulation, abdominal organs, ovaries and prostate. It can help

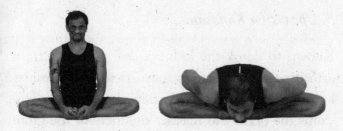

relieve problems ranging from piles, hypertension, menstrual discomfort to sciatica and even alleviate symptoms of menopause. Consistently doing this while pregnant has been known to ease childbirth.

Method:
- Sit in Dandasana and breathe ten times.
- Then bring your feet together, soles touching. Draw your heels into your pelvis, fold both legs to the side and grabbing your feet from the top, open your with both hands.
- Exhale, touch head to the floor, bending from the lower back, not the neck. If you can't reach the floor, stay wherever you can.
- Breathe five times. Don't worry if your knees don't touch the floor. Don't push your knees to the ground, instead open your inner thighs turning them outwards. As you continue to practise this posture and others, your hips will open up.
- Breathe five times.
- Inhale, lift the head up. Exhale.

5. *Upavistha Konasana*

Known to detox the kidneys and ease pain from arthritis and sciatica, this asana stretches the insides and back of the legs and strengthens hamstrings, calms the brain and releases tightness of the groin and inner thighs.

This asana is also very beneficial for pregnant women. It aids labour, relaxes muscles and helps women gain flexibility to stretch and deliver with ease. This must be practised during pregnancy to increase a pregnant woman's pelvic floor area.

Method:

- Sit on the floor and spread your legs wide. Sit up straight with your spine.
- Catch your heels with your hands and lift your head up. Exhale, and touch your chin to the floor. For those who can't reach their knees or can't touch their chin or forehead to the floor, you can bend your knees slightly.
- Breathe five times.
- Inhale, head up, look up.
- Exhale, release.

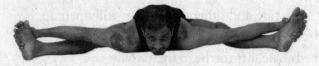

6. Supta Padangusthasana

A restorative asana, Supta Padangusthasana is for those suffering from lower back pain. This asana stretches your hamstrings and therefore your lower back without excessively straining your spine. It increases flexibility in the hips, strengthens the lower abdomen. This asana is also very good for pregnant women, as it can aid in a faster and painless delivery, by opening up the pelvic and hip muscles.

Method:
- Lie down, exhale.
- Inhale, catch your right big toe with your right hand. Your left leg remains on the ground. Keep both legs straight. Bend your knee slightly if you can't catch your big toe with a straightened leg.
- Exhale, touch your chin to your knee or bring your head as close to your leg as you can.
- Breathe five times.
- Inhale and exhale, lower your head to the floor.
- Take your right leg to the right side and look on the left. Breathe five times.
- Inhale, bring your right leg back to the centre.
- Exhale, touch your chin to your knee.
- Inhale, lower your head to the floor.

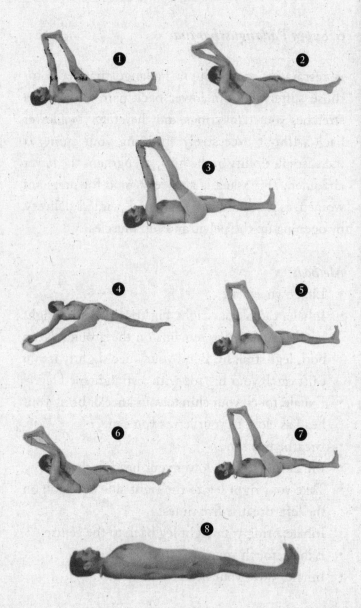

- Exhale, release your right toe and lower your right leg to the floor.

Pavanmuktasana

A variation of Supta Padangusthasana, Pavanmuktasana is excellent to ease gastric problems. Pavanmukta means release of air.

Method:

While lying on your back instead of catching your toes, bend your legs and catch your feet with both hands, each hand holding it's corresponding foot from the outer edge of the foot. Alternatively bend one leg and catch your knee from behind, to pull your knee towards your head.

Do this five times on each side.

7. Utthita Hasta Padangusthasana

This intermediate balancing pose is one of the tougher ones in Ashtanga's standing sequence. Translated to mean extended hand-to-big toe, this asana brings grounding and a growth from within that infuses your life with stability. Utthita Hasta Padangusthasana is used to develop our sense of balance and concentration. It helps strengthen ankles, thighs, calves and the lower abdomen, stretches hamstrings and opens out hips and shoulders.

Method:

- Stand straight in Samasthitih, exhale.
- Inhale, lift your right leg up and catch your right big toe with your right hand. Keep both legs as straight as possible.
- Exhale, touch the chin to the knees. If you can't reach your knee with your head, lower yourself bending from the lower back, till wherever is comfortable. Initially bending at the knees helps with balance. But keep trying to straighten your legs out as that strengthens your leg muscles and your core. Keep your left hand on your waist and push down through your left foot, grounding yourself.
- Breathe five times.

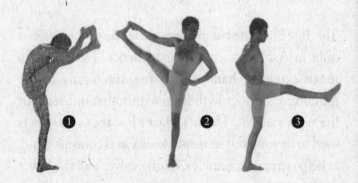

- Inhale and take your leg out to the right, and look towards the left if you can. Your chin is over your shoulder. Breathe five times.
- Inhale, bring your leg back to the front.
- Exhale, touch your chin to your knee. Or lower your head as far down as you can.
- Inhale, lift the head. Place both hands on the waist. Breathe five times with your leg lifted up, straight in front of you, toes pointing out.
- Exhale release and return to Samasthitih.
- Inhale, lift your left leg up and catch your left big toe with your left hand. Keep both legs as straight as possible.
- Exhale, touch the chin to the knee. If you can't reach your knee with your head, lower yourself bending from the lower back, till wherever is comfortable. Initially bending at the knees helps with balance. But keep trying to straighten your legs out as that strengthens your leg muscles and your core. Keep your left hand on your waist and push down through your left foot, grounding yourself.
- Breathe five times.
- Inhale and take your leg out to the right, and look towards the left if you can. Your chin is over your shoulder. Breathe five times.
- Inhale, bring your leg back to the front.

- Exhale, touch your chin to your knee. Or lower your head as far down as you can.
- Inhale, lift the head. Place both hands on the waist. Breathe five times with your leg lifted up, straight in front of you, toes pointing out.
- Exhale, release and return to Samasthitih.

Note: Bend your knees if you find it tough to straighten your legs. Or you can support yourself against a wall if you find it tough to balance.

8. *Utkatasana*

Utkata means powerful. This fierce posture looks easy but is tough on your legs, arms and back, strengthening and stretching all three. It also works on your hip flexors, ankles and calves, and is a good opening for your chest and shoulders. Utkatasana stimulates abdominal organs and builds endurance.

Method:
- Stand in Samasthitih.
- Inhale and raise your arms perpendicular to the floor. Keep the arms parallel, palms facing inwards and exhale as you bend your knees. Keep your thighs as parallel as possible to the floor. Imagine

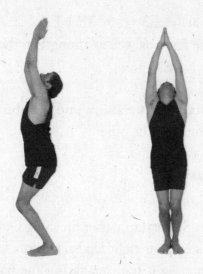

you are sitting on a chair, as you go deeper. May sure your back stays straight and you don't collapse in the lower back. Shoulders should stay down, far from the ears.
• Take five breaths slowly and come up, release.

9. *Virabhadrasana 1 and 2*

Virabhadra is the ferocious warrior incarnation of Shiva, often seen with many arms and a garland of skulls. Warrior postures are for strength, confidence and stability. These two asanas strengthen the lower back, arms and legs while stretching the chest, lungs, shoulders, belly and groin. They help ease arthritic pains in the knee, as well as strengthen the muscles around the knee.

Note: Practice Utkatasana and Virabhadrasana together one after the other.

Virabhadrasana 1

Method:

- Stand in Samasthitih after finishing Utkatasana.
- Inhale, step your right leg back into a low lunge. Turn your right foot out facing the back. Bend from your right knee.
- Your left foot is slightly turned in. Lift your arms above your head, palms together and look up if you can at your thumbs. Your right knee should be above your right ankle. Relax your shoulders and

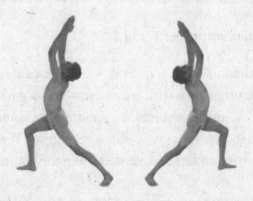

stretch from your spine. Take five breaths slowly. If you can't look up then look in front. Keep your back straight.

- Inhale, come up, turn your right foot in and left foot out towards the front of your mat.
- Exhale, bend from your left knee. Your left knee should be above your left ankle. Relax your shoulders and stretch from your spine. Take five breaths slowly. If you can't look up then look n front. Keep your back straight.
- Inhale, step forward. Exhale to Samasthitih.

Virabhadrasana 2

Method:

- From Samasthitih, inhale and step your right foot back. With your right foot out and toes pointing straight, keep your left foot perpendicular to your front foot, and release into a low lunge.
- Lift your arms up parallel to the ground, with your palms facing down towards the floor. Keep your right knee above your right ankle and your wrists in line with your shoulders. Gaze at your right middle finger, relax your shoulders, dropping them from your ears. Take five breaths slowly.
- Inhale, turn around to the front of your mat. Now your right foot is out, toes pointing straight ahead

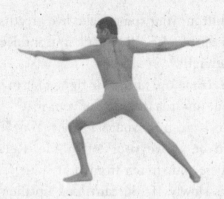

and your right foot is behind you and perpendicular to the foot in front. Lift your arms up parallel to the ground, with your palms facing down towards the floor. Release into a low lunge. Keep your left knee above your left ankle and your wrists in line with your shoulders. Gaze at your left middle finger, relax your shoulders, dropping them from your ears. Take five breaths slowly.

- Inhale, step forward. Exhale to Samasthitih.

10. Urdhva Dhanurasana

This is an advanced posture so please practise it carefully. Urdhva Dhanurasana stimulates your pituitary and thyroid glands, strengthens the spinal cord, legs, buttocks, wrists, arms and vertebrae, whilst also giving your stomach, lungs and thorax an intense stretch. It relieves lower back pain, stress, depression and even asthma.

Both the full asana and a modified Urdhva Dhanurasana are good for cardiovascular problems. This posture clears blocked arteries, and gets the blood flowing.

Note: Always warm up before this posture. Setu Bandha Sarvangasana is a wonderful asana to help you come into full Urdhva Dhanurasana. Avoid if you have wrist or neck issues, or suffer from high or low blood pressure.

Method:
- Lie down on the floor with your knees bent and feet hip-width apart.

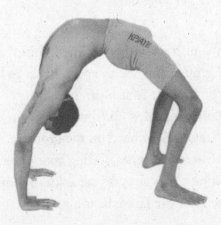

- Bend your elbows and place your palms on the floor near your ears with your fingers facing your shoulders.
- Inhale, lift your hips up first. Then press into your palms and push away from the floor, as you exhale. If this is tough, first come on to the crown of your head. Do not let your elbows or your knees fall outwards. Rotate your shoulders outwards and your thighs inwards. Take five breaths slowly.
- To release, exhale and bring your shoulders, neck and head down slowly, chin to chest. Avoid landing on your head.

An equally effective modification for Urdhva Dhanurasana is Setu Bandha Sarvangasana.

Setu Bandha Sarvangasana

Method:
- Lie on your back with your knees folded and feet on the ground hip-width apart. Place your hands palms down near your hips.
- Inhale, lift your hips up. Your chin is tucked into your chest, back of head on the ground.
- Breathe here five times, feeling your chest expand and contract. You can grab your ankles if comfortable.
- Release after the last exhalation.

11. *Padmasana*

This asana is named after the lotus for its resemblance both physically and metaphorically with the flower that grows from the mud. Patanjali in the Yoga Sutras talks about finding stillness and comfort to be able to meditate or perform any asana. Both *Yoga Yagnavalkya* and *Yoga Vasistha* state that Padmasana destroys not just disease of the body, but great sins too.

Padmasana is therefore the greatest and best of all asanas, easy to practice and should be performed by all.[5]

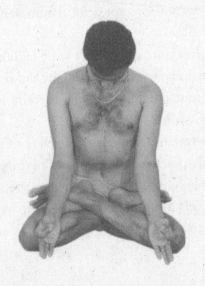

This asana helps cure flatulence because of the pressure your heels apply on your organs in and around the stomach region. The posture is also used for dhyana, meditation and pranayama. Sitting in Padmasana and forward bending will activate your jathra agni, as well as your respiratory organs. This asana can even cure insomnia caused by irregular breathing patterns.

Method:
- Sit on the floor and try to take your right foot on top of your left thigh and your left foot on to your right thigh.
- If you cannot attempt a full Padmasana, do one leg at a time.
- Straighten your spine, tuck your tailbone in and breathe. Keep your spine straight and breath. This opens your chest and lungs, thereby increasing oxygen intake.
- Initially you may find it hard to practice Padmasana, but daily practice will help you increase the time you can hold your posture. When you bend forward both heels should be pressing into your lower abdomen and thighs.

Highlighted below are the problems and the asanas that cure them:

1. Backaches – lower and upper back pain:

- Utthita Trikonasana builds strength in the legs and back, while increasing flexibility. Stretches hamstrings and strengthens the abdomen.
- Pachimattasana stretches the spine, and creates the desired gaps between your vertebrae.
- Upavistha Konasana stretches the hamstrings and strengthens the abdomen and makes the spine stronger. Can help sciatica pain.
- Supta Padangusthasana for the lower back.
- Utthita Hasta Padangusthasana strengthens the back.
- Utkatasana builds strength.

2. Flatulence and indigestion

- Utthita Trikonasana relives stomach pain from indigestion.
- Upavistha Konasana stimulates the abdominal organs and the kidney for detox.
- Pavanmuktasana almost immediately relieves discomfort from flatulence.
- Pachimattasana improves digestion.
- Padmasana relieves gas and bloating.

3. Headaches

- Pachimattasana can reduce migraine pain.
- Padmasana helps you meditate to reduce headaches.
- Adho Mukha Svanasana helps circulate blood in the head and back of the neck area.

4. Respiratory problems

- Virabhadrasana 1 and 2 are upward stretches that expand lungs to aid breathing.
- Urdhva Dhanurasana is an intense expansion of the lungs to aid breathing.

5. Erratic or painful periods and menopause

- Utthita Trikonasana stimulates the ovaries, stretches the abdominal muscles, and helps relieve menopause symptoms.
- Pachimattasana stimulates the ovaries, and helps alleviate menopause pains.
- Baddha Konasana reduces menstrual pain.

6. Anxiety and insomnia

- Pachimattasana reduces stress, anxiety and even panic attacks.
- Upavistha Konasana is very calming.
- Baddha Konasana eases fatigue.

- Urdhva Dhanurasana opens your heart to the universe.
- Padmasana is great for meditation.

7. High and low blood pressure
- Pachimattasana is a stress reliever and normalizes blood pressure.
- Baddha Konasana improves blood circulation and reduces hypertension.

8. Prostate problems

- Baddha Konasana stimulates the abdominal organs, improving prostate health.

9. Hamstrings and calves

- Supta Padangusthasana opens up the lower back and stretches the hamstrings without injuring the back.
- Utthita Trikonasana is an intense side stretch.
- Upavistha Konasana is an intense stretch for the groin, inner thighs, all the way down to the ankles.
- Utthita Hasta Padangusthasana helps stretch and balance from within.
- Utkatasana strengthens calves.

10. Overall strength

- Utkatasana is a strong squat.
- Upavistha Konasana builds up calves and thigh muscles.
- Utthita Hasta Padangusthasana creates a core strong enough to stand and stretch and improves balance.
- Virabhadrasana 1 and 2 builds warrior-like body strength.
- Urdhva Dhanurasana strengthens the thighs and lower back for a deeper lift.

~

- Warm up, strengthen and stretch your body with the Surya Namaskara routine.
- Baddha Konasana is a powerful healer for men and women.
- Keep your breathing strong and steady throughout your practice, as vinyasa brings a healing heat to your body.
- Sitting in Padmasana is not just meditative, but by activating your Jathra Agni it also cures digestive problems.

6

Deeper Breaths Result in a Longer Life

In his book, *Autobiography of a Yogi*, Paramahansa Yogananda reveals an interesting bit of information. He says that those species that breathe slowly, live the longest.

Turtles take four to five breaths a minute and live for hundreds of years.

Cats and dogs who breathe many more times a second than us, live a decade or two.

Humanbeings inhale and exhale 21,600 times a day, in a resting state, so we fall inbetween these two species.

This may sound like a tenuous argument, but hear me out.

When you have good breathing habits, you take in more oxygen, which results in optimal brain function. Brain cells need a continuous supply of oxygen to work. Case in point: after spending an entire day in the editing room where you have been editing your film, you find yourself feeling sleepy and sluggish and even perhaps anxious. That's because of the excess carbondioxide you have been breathing in. And as soon as you step out of the room, you're markedly more refreshed.

It's no surprise that when the brain has an adequate oxygen supply, you're less stressed, more active and energetic and more at peace. This in turn means less work for your heart and mind. A stress-free life has a direct connection with longevity. When we live without anxiety, our bodies are not burdened with cortisol, the stress hormone. And so we function on a relaxed system that works efficiently and at optimum levels.

But how many of us actually live without stress? Our modern lifestyles, for most of us, are characterized by umpteen daily stresses - work, deadlines, financial pressures, emotional triggers, abuse, even traffic. The list is endless. Instinctively our physiological reactions to stress cause shallow heart rate and irregular breathing, leading us to use less than 20 per cent of our lung capacity. All this affects our well-being.

Breathing slowly, consciously and with attention helps us improve lung capacity. Almost the same way exercise does. It delivers more oxygen into our bodies. This kind of conscious breathing can help improve overall health, mood, energy and sleep. It helps us live longer. The *Hatha Yoga Pradipika* states that when the breath wanders, and is irregular, the mind is also unsteady, but when the breath is still, so is the mind, and the yogi lives long. So one should restrain the breath.

However, slow, deep, mindful breathing from the lungs takes a little work and awareness. This is where the ancient technique of pranayama can help you. Pranayama is an ancient practice that dates back centuries. Patanjali in the Yoga Sutras says that if done properly pranayama can help alleviate the darkness of ignorance, affliction and karma. And from there emerges the light of clarity.

The word 'prana' means life force and the 'ayama' means to draw it out. Doing pranayama releases emotional blocks in your body, letting prana flow uninhibited.

Pranayama to control the mind

Guruji would often say, 'Ashtanga practice is a breathing practice . . . the rest is just bending.' And how right he is. The yoga method according to my grandfather meant that you first perfected asana and then perfected pranayama. The pranayama techniques we practice are meant to extend your breathing.

Nadi shodhana and Ujjayi pranayama are two powerful breathing techniques that help regulate our prana and apana. The Bhagavad Gita says that steadying the flow of prana (incoming breath) and apana (outgoing breath) helps control our sense organs and the mind. Prana and apana must be equal. If you inhale for two seconds, your exhalations should also be for two seconds.

Ashtanga focuses heavily on breathing. Prana is centred in the third eye. It flows from the nostrils to the heart. Apana is energy that flows upwards from the pelvic region. It regulates elimination and diseases of the lower abdomen, kidney, urinary tract and intestines. 'Just as a lion, elephant or tiger may be gradually brought under control, so must prana be correctly attended to, otherwise, it destroys the practitioner,' Guruji quotes from the *Hatha Yoga*

Pradipika in *Yoga Mala*. I would like to share with you a yogi's breathing practices that can help reduce the number of breaths we take in a day, thus increasing our lifespan.

Why you should adopt a pranayama practice

I have seen pranayama cure people of all kinds of blockages in their nostrils, allergies, asthma, bronchitis and congestion in the lungs. Pranayama breathing techniques can fight dust and plant allergies and cleanse our systems and lungs from toxic pollutants.

In large gatherings, we often end up breathing in other people's toxins. Their bacteria enters our body making us sick. Pranayama counters these toxins.

People who get breathless from climbing stairs or walking at a brisk pace can develop their lung capacity with pranayama. Those who find they hyperventilate or become breathless in moments of stress, emotional instability and anxiety can calm themselves with these deep breathing techniques. Deep breathing helps increase concentration and is even prescribed for children diagnosed with ADHD and other attention disorders.

A simple twenty-minute routine every morning

reduces stress and anxieties and can help you welcome the day joyfully.

Unlike the shat kriyas we learned about in the detox chapter, pranayama is essential to a yogi's asana practice. Ashtanga practitioners end each asana practice with a routine of breathing exercises. The very word hatha (the foundations of all yoga) is broken down as 'ha' meaning Surya Nadi (inhalations through right nostril) and 'tha' meaning Chandra Nadi (breathing through left nostril). Controlling prana as it moves through each nadi (nose) is called Hatha Yoga. This helps keep your blood pressure low, improves your concentration and keeps you calm the entire day, even through moments of anxiety and stress.

Nadi shodhana pranayama or alternate nostril breathing

Nadi shodhana breathing gives you the tools to deal with anxiety, insomnia and work and life stress. Even road rage can be lowered with this practice. Other issues that come from anxiety and stress such as high blood pressure, depression and anxiety can be alleviated if you can commit to these practices for three to four months. When you deal with moments of stress with a calm mind and steady breathing, you will see how the world around you changes.

Nadi shodhana or alternate nostril breathing is a simple and powerful breathing practice. The best time to practise it is early morning, on an empty stomach. If you don't have a regular asana practice, find time during the morning or at night to practise pranayama. Ensure at least a forty-five minute gap after a meal, before doing nadi shodhana.

The duration of your inhalation and exhalation must be the same. Do three sets of Nadi shodhana in about five minutes.

Method:
- Sit in Padmasana or cross-legged, whatever is comfortable. Take a few deep breaths.
- Fold your index and middle fingers of the right hand to the base of your thumb. Press into the side of your right nostril towards the bottom of the nostril, and inhale completely through your left nostril. Don't force yourself. Make your inhalation easy and free.
- Now release your thumb and press down your left nostril with the tips of your little and ring fingers and exhale from the right nostril.
- Then press down the thumb on the right nostril

again and inhale from the left. Repeat five times, and switch sides.

- Now press down on the left nostril with your little and ring fingers, and inhale through the right nostril.
- Then press down with your thumb on your right nostril and exhale through the left, and then inhale through the right nostril.
- Repeat this five times.

Ujjai breathing

Ujjayi breathing sounds like the calming waves of the ocean. It has a magical and immediate calming effect on me whenever I practise it. Ujjayi breathing is also very similar to what we use in our asana practice. It is the breath that correlates to each movement or asana. This symbiosis between breath and movement creates strong prana within us, and is a powerful cure for many health issues.

Practise five minutes of three sets of inhalation and exhalation for benefits. This is not a replacement for medicines prescribed by a doctor for medical conditions such as blood pressure or cholesterol. These are preventive and can supplement any treatment one may undergo.

Method:
- Sit in Padmasana.
- Inhale, taking air into your belly in a deep, audible manner, with a little bit of force. But not too much. Feel your stomach contracting. And then exhale all that air out, and feel your stomach expanding.
- Extend your inhalations from a second to two and then even more. You are aiming for long inhalations and equally long exhalations, by extending your prana and asana.

Meditation increases your lifespan

According to the shastras, we have six enemies or arishadvargas (delusions) within each one of us. Our true nature, our antar atman, is untouched by these delusions. These are:

Kama: lust
Krodha: anger
Madha: pride
Matsariya: jealousy
Lobha: greed
Moha: attraction

The spiritual goal post we are moving towards is realization of that antar atman, the supreme soul.

153

I often think of this inner soul as a pure pearl in an oyster shell. To get to the pearl you have to get rid of the shell. The shell is layered with delusions or Arishadvargas. And once we get rid of that shell we gain complete clarity of spiritual knowledge and realization of the antar atman.

For those who aren't scholars of philosophy this may sound absurd, but what I am coming to is the concept we are all quite familiar with – that of meditation or as we in the Ashtanga world know it, dhyana. Let me explain to you what dhayana is and why I don't like to use the word mediation.

In the Yoga Sutras, Patanjali says '*yogas citta vritti nirodhah*'. When you are in a state of yoga all misconceptions (vritti) disappear. To go deeper into our practice and be focused in everyday life we need to overcome chitta vriti or monkey chatter or mind chatter. That's the voice in your mind that is constantly doing lists, second-guessing you, telling you the grass is greener on the other side.

In fact it was Buddha who described the human mind like a screeching, chattering, monkey swinging from branch to branch, hard to control. That's where dhyana, meditation or contemplation comes in. The West has only now caught up with the concept of meditation, but 'dhyana' comes from schools of Vedanta from 1500 BCE. Dhyana is what leads to samadhi – the culmination where the mind is totally still, where we can tap into our inner atma or our inner soul.

Dhyana is the method by which you focus your attention on an object or at one place and meditate so you can stop disturbances of the mind. Dhyana helps bring your mind to a still and quiet place. Meditation is not separate from your yoga practice.

An Ohio State University study published in *Social Psychological and Personality Science* found people who are affiliated to religious organizations and practise abstinence and meditation live longer by about five years. The sense of community one finds during spiritual practices and the quietness and stress-abating effects of meditation and prayer are very strong. Being quiet fosters connections within you.

For me, spirituality is about being a good human being. And this automatically leads to a life of less conflict, both internally and externally. Spirituality is not born of religion. When big religious institutions get caught up in politics, it divides people. We are all humanbeings with the same capacity to love and pray. Spiritual practices tap into that and guide us on how to conduct ourselves. We start to think about our actions, reactions and thoughts. When we aren't caught up in the six enemies, we can get clarity on what we are. Our actions become pure. And then we can think of ourselves as being spiritual.

As you search, you crave that which you did not know. Your spiritual endeavours help you to not get caught up in samsara, what Shankaracharya called the cycle of birth and death. Thus, you can break the cycle of karma. There are three kinds of karma. Sanchitta karma, that which we accumulate from our previous births, prarabdha karma, that which you accumulate in this life and agami, the future consequences of present actions. To get rid of suffering and the cycle of karma is to have a proper spiritual knowledge. Therefore spirituality simply means ridding oneself of arishadvargas or delusions.

How to meditate

Trataka
Ever been excessively distracted and felt your eyes flit here and there almost out of your control. If yes, you will recognize the importance of stillness of the eyes and how that in turn leads to stillness of the mind. Trataka helps weak eyes and can even alleviate headaches, as it works to strengthen your eye muscles.

Place a dot about eight to ten feet away. Shut out thoughts, empty your mind. Bring your gaze or drishti to one point – the dot or flame of a candle – to quell distractions in your mind. In kriya, this is called trataka, where you focus on a dot without blinking, until you get tears.

Japa

Doing japa is different from trataka where you focus from the outside.

Sit still, cross-legged with your eyes closed, for about eight minutes and focus on whatever deity you feel connected with. Chanting or practising japa also helps generate energies. When you chant you create vibrations by moving your tongue in repetition. Don't forget to continue breathing through your mouth while chanting. Chanting strengthens your lungs.

What you chant doesn't have to be connected with religion. You can choose any japa that you are comfortable with, that has been given to you by your family or a guru. Chanting Om represents universal energy, and is a simple and powerful place to start.

~

Ultimately, at the risk of sounding like a broken record, I come back to the same thing. To sit still, focus for long periods of time you need a strong body and healthy, disease-free organs. So every meditative practice is made more effective if you have strong asana practice.

We may not want to live for hundreds of years, but we can take a leaf from the grand turtle's book and try to slow down. Try these breathing and meditation techniques and see how your instinctive reactions become so much more measured and intelligent.

~

- Breath slowly to improve lung capacity, find calm in moments of stress and increase longevity.
- Practising pranayama cures allergies, helps us control our mind and releases emotional blocks in the body.
- Chant to connect with the universal energy and heal through auditory vibrations.
- Meditate to still your eyes, and in turn still your mind.

7

Help Others to Help Yourself

During my childhood, we lived next door to a man who was a Sanskrit scholar. We were sent to him to study shlokas, the Upanishads and the Bhagavad Gita. All very heavy subjects for children! But my cousins and I loved him. He taught us in a manner that made even these ancient texts of philosophy and literature very interesting. He would make us enact parts of the epics (you know how much I love a good Hanuman story), we would go on walks and explore the outdoors while reciting shlokas, and one summer when we were eleven years old he enlisted my cousins and me as volunteers at a Rashtriya Swayamsevak Sangh camp in Mysore.

At the camp they had talks, training in various

subjects from music to morals, we were taught martial arts, did physical training, enlisted in community service to clean the parks and roads. I was introduced to the idea of a Swachh Bharat long before the term had been coined.

The atmosphere at the camp was spiritual. The camp leaders taught us stories about Hanuman that stayed with me for life. One of my favourites is from the Ramayana when Lakshman falls unconscious in battle, gravely injured by an arrow shot by Ravana's son, Indrajit. He didn't have more than a day to live. Hanuman approached the Sri Lankan royal physician Sushena for guidance. He told Hanuman to bring the herb sanjeevani to heal Lakshman, from Mount Dronagiri, one of the highest peaks of the mighty Himalayas. A herb so powerful it can cure the most serious of nervous system problems. To spot it Hanuman had to look for a plant that emitted a light.

And so Hanuman leapt over oceans, and flew over vast expanses of land to the Himalayas. Unfortunately all his strength and speed weren't going to help Hanuman because when he reached the mighty mountain range, the not very medically trained monkey god could not identify this powerful medicinal herb. Even today, scientists and researchers are trying to find this elusive herb. When Hanuman couldn't find the herb, he decided to bring the entire mountain back, thus most iconic images of Hanuman are of him carrying Mount Dronagiri. The story of Hanuman lifting Dronagiri inspires me during challenging times. On his way back, the sun started to rise, so Hanuman decided to capture the sun under his arm so that he could arrive with the medicine the same day. I love that image of the monkey god with the sun under his arm, symbolizing positivity and perseverance – just grab the sun and run towards your problems!

Besides all the stories and spiritual guidance at the camp, there was a lot of emphasis on seva or service, the importance of being selfless, of selfless action and how one should always help people in difficulty. The ideas appealed to me and even though I was young, I knew I wanted to do something special for my community. But it took me a while to understand the magic behind seva, or selfless service. Being ageless is intricately intertwined with self-lessness. And it's a rather simple logic.

Each one of us is under some kind of stress on a daily basis. Life has become more competitive, and there's little we can do about external stresses. Think about the questions that beset you in just one hour: Will I make it to my meeting on time? Where will I get the money to pay off my loan? What will I eat for lunch? Why does she not respond to my emails?

Now, pay close attention to these stresses. What do you notice?

The answer is: I.

We are the creator and cause of all our anxieties! Isn't this just madness?

So it only makes sense to take the focus away from yourself. By this, I'm not asking you to forget about your well-being. What I'm suggesting is to take time out of your schedule to engage with your community or by volunteering in a service that is about others. It doesn't even have to be a formal affair. Help out a relative or a neighbour if you prefer. By engaging in selfless service you'll find yourself less worried and consumed with yourself. And this takes away some load off your shoulders. Remember, thinking about and helping others takes the focus away from your own problems. And in a strange but simple way, you will be doing yourself a favour, both emotionally and physically, because excessive stress is linked to a host of lifestyle-related diseases like obesity, blood pressure, insomnia, among others.

Social connectedness

In 2003, I read about journalist Dan Buettner's 'blue zones', which resonated with me deeply.

The blue zones included the island of Sardinia in Italy, Okinawa in Japan, Loma Linda in California, Costa Rica's Nicoya Peninsula and Ikaria, a remote Greek island. Each place was a long way from the other, but they shared something in common – these were the healthiest in the world where women and men lived to a hundred years or more. People lived not just longer, but healthier lives, free from disease and chronic conditions.

Each city, town or island had its own specific reason for such marvellous figures of longevity, but the common ones included diets heavy in locally available plants and legumes and moderate exercise.

But there was one factor that stood out for me – social connectedness. People living in the blue zones have access to excellent support systems. They are involved in their community. This is an important factor in longevity.

While religion and faith provided strong communities to the people of these regions, and a foundation through which they could give back, another commonality was putting family first, living in close proximity to parents, committing to one life partner and investing love and time in their children. Being connected with your community has been proven to reduce stress, depression and addictions, which in turn aids longevity.[1] Think of how many times a spouse has helped you kick a bad habit, or a friend has provided you with support in a difficult time, or a relative has given you advice for your budding business. Think also of a restaurant where joyful chatter is the predominant sound, not the ping-ing of cellphone notifications. Family gatherings, while potentially chaotic and sometimes even contentious, make us feel wanted and provide us with a sense of belonging. When a family member puts everything on hold to be by your side during times of sorrow and even joy, does that kinship not make you feel unburdened and ready to face the world? Human beings cannot function in isolation, as islands, and we should not forget that in our race to get ahead.

In India, we once had a strong support system – the joint family. But today that network is disintegrating. I mourn the loss of the sense of community from the days when we lived in joint families and depended on the support and love of our neighbours and our villages. We lived with a sense of belonging born from real connections we had with people around us. And we knew that we would never have to deal with our problems alone.

Today, our lives are far removed from that. We have isolated, island-like existences. Our only connections are on the internet with people who we rarely see in real life. When we remove that sense of responsibility to our community, we become defined in terms of winning over everyone else, no matter what it takes. We become focused on power and are enveloped by selfishness. When we are unhappy or dissatisfied with our lives, we lose the ability to untangle ourselves from multiple layers of negativity. We become defined by the emotions that take over all logical thinking and lead to further anxieties and insecurities.

One way to get out of this cycle of harmful negativity is to shift the focus away from our troubles and make someone happy by giving them our time and attention. Doing this helps us realize there are entire communities that can benefit from our knowledge and experiences that we may have invested a lot of time and money into, that we can pass on for free. And in the bargain take the attention away from ourselves.

There is an ugly self-obsession that has reared its head in the form of the loudness of social media. I often talk about social media in my conferences. When our minds are constantly filled with the chatter and the opinions of social media networks we give stillness no opportunity to thrive.

We become so obsessed with the perfect picture we present to the world (read that to mean social media) of our lives, of our work, of our yoga, that we become frustrated when we realize that this artificially created story does not exist. By breaking away from these unhealthy obsessions we can steer away from the stresses of the fast lane and the fake constructs of life shown on the internet. Think of it this way – a picture may be worth a thousand words, but half of those words are from the photographer and subject and the other half are the viewers'. So, whenever we feel upset that our friend's life seems so much more joyful, successful or exciting than ours, we must remember that the expectations and failures are ours.

Once we step away from this myopic, dysfunctional way of viewing the world we can start to make space for the people around us in a more fulfilling manner. What I have been leading up to is the wonderful concept of seva. In India, we are lucky to have been initiated into seva early on, as each one of our religions actively encourages the method of worship through service to the community.

These selfless acts have been written about in great detail in the Bhagavad Gita and the Quran. Altruistic Sikhs everywhere have made the world a much better place thanks to their concept of seva as taught in the Guru Granth Sahib. Over 100,000 people are fed every day at the Golden Temple. The number increases on weekends and festivals. In Islam, Sadaqah is a concept of giving that literally calls for people to give from their possessions. The Quran says, '…And whoever volunteers good – then indeed, Allah is appreciative and Knowing.'

For those who are wondering where to begin, I have tried in my own humble way to explain what kind of seva I partake in. Maybe this can help you create a blueprint for your own seva.

Seva from guru to shishya

I often wonder why KPJAYI needed to become such a large institution. When we started, our goal was to gain deeper knowledge, it was never wealth or fame. But I realized this knowledge was given to us to be shared with more and more people. This is what comes with this practice. You have to balance your own sadhana with teaching.

Being a yogi, you aren't just giving your students asanas, you are also giving them guidance. That's your seva to them.

Seva for yourself: Since the time I was a child I have felt a deep connect with nature and wildlife. Growing up, we would visit the Kabini National Park often.

And in 2005 my family and I visited Africa. I took some photographs of wildlife in their natural habitat and fell in love with photography. I had to be careful not to get too attached or too addicted. People around me will always have better photographic equipment than me, and do more trips than me, but I realized early on that I would not be able to pursue photography very often, so kept my equipment minimal.

I feel that my love for photography is somewhere connected to the age-old relationship yoga has with nature. Mayurasana, Matsyasana and Kurmasana are just some of the asanas that have come from rishis and munis, ancient saints who sat in the forest watching nature in all its glory and wonder and doing their sadhana. Here they conducted their own research to help people live a peaceful, happy and harmonious life with each other and with other animals and trees.

The deepest connections need to be with flora and fauna. The only way forward is by remembering asana is just one facet of being a yoga practitioner.

Seva for nature: Being a yogi means you have to think about how you live among animals and nature. All living beings have the same rights. Cutting just one tree destroys the habitat of hundreds of living things. We can't live our lives thinking only about what we can take from nature, and how we can use her for monetary gains.

We recently planted around 200 trees as our seva to nature. With the amount of pollution in our cities, urban yogis need to think about planting trees, and how this affects their yoga practice too. Instead of visiting temples just start by being kind to the animals and trees around you. We have to ensure our children have fresh, oxygen-laden air to breathe. I always tell my students if you have a child, plant ten trees. Then your children can grow with the trees. They will develop an important connection with mother earth.

A child who plants trees, learns about nature and the importance of trees and contributing to the earth. No one has time to stop, sit and take in nature these days. When you plant a tree, you grow with that tree.

It's like looking after a child. You develop a connection with nature. Research has shown that just a few hours in fresh air increases people's energy by 90 per cent, making them feel more alive and energetic and increases their resilience to physical illness.[2]

It has also been proven scientifically that when you are in a clean room where oxygen levels are high your brain activity increases by 30 per cent. Children who are in a clean room for an exam do phenomenally better.

Pranayama, that essential limb of yoga we have already learned about, means breath control. It's about controlling your breath to expel toxins and infuse vital life back into your body. But any yoga done in unclean air, where there is a lack of oxygen, will not grant you a calm mind. Remember to practise yoga and pranayama in a room with clean air.

Yogis escape to forests and mountains because when fresh air reaches your brain you become healthy. Toxic air disturbs your mind. Practising in urban cities can be detrimental to your yoga. Clean, fresh air is very important for one's practice.

Upon entering a forest you automatically feel more alive. You feel a difference with the excess of oxygen that goes straight to your brain and your body. You feel bright, awakened and almost enlightened.

Plant trees around your property or your home that are indigenous. Decorative trees are of no use as they are usually alien to local geographical conditions. I have recommended to many people who have breathing issues or even psychological problems, such as depression, to regularly visit parks, and to breathe there and just soak in nature. It's truly the best cure.

Seva for your country: When it comes to your country, start small. Be honest. Pay your taxes, follow the rules and be a responsible citizen. This is the seva that will help your country improve. At KPJAYI we don't take any grants. We pay taxes honestly and ask for no income tax exemptions. We give 40 to 45 per cent of our earnings to the government to help the leaders of our country do seva on a large scale.

Seva for your community: In the Bhagavad Gita, Lord Krishna tells Arjuna that just like yajnas are performed for the rain gods to make rain which in turn produces food or yields a good crop, people must also perform selfless acts for communities to perform at their best capacity. Here food is just a metaphor, not actual financial gains.

A real yogi considers everyone to be equal. A real yogi shares money and knowledge. A real yogi helps uplift people. A real yogi helps others progress. As you practise yoga these thoughts will come to you. At the shala we have scholarships for Indian students who can't afford to pay the fees. In India we have lost a connection with traditional yoga. Today there is an urgent need to connect with Indians. Indians are inherently spiritual, and by practising Ashtanga Yoga we can easily grasp concepts of spirituality and work towards being more yogic. But we need to be dedicated. Teachers also need to encourage students to be dedicated. They could hold free classes to encourage people to take up yoga.

To illustrate this bear with me while I tell you a little story from a conference in Bengaluru. On day one there were only foreign participants and I told the organizers that yoga was for everyone and we must give everyone a chance to learn. On the second day about three hundred locals who had never experienced Ashtanga Yoga in their lives came to the conference. On the third day students were crying, they said they had no idea a yoga practice like this existed where there was such a strong focus on breath and movement. They loved it. Only when you do the practice will you realize the beauty of it. You will realize the beauty of the method and its power. This is my seva.

Seva at office and school: Each one of us should donate a part of our earnings to a well-recognized charity. Do proper research on how the charity spends the money that comes to it. If you work for a big corporate collect money and try to use it directly to help people.

Yoga should be introduced in corporate and public offices and in schools. It's very important for children to be encouraged to practise yoga from a very young age. Children these days are easily distracted and need to be focused on things other than blue screens. They need to get exercise.

In government and private offices and at universities, people can start with a simple asana practice and breathing exercises. This is what will make us more productive as a nation. These are the routines that will help people live harmoniously, and bring peace to our communities on a micro level and the world on a macro level.

Quiet seva: Always do seva quietly. In Kannada we have a saying, which translates roughly to, when you do something with your right hand, your left hand shouldn't know you've done it. Unfortunately, people do seva for publicity. This is not real seva. We give schoolbags to over a thousand children every year, we plant hundreds of trees every year and we rarely talk about it.

~

Islam, Sikhism, Buddhism and Hinduism are just some of the religions that emphasize on concepts of seva. Besides what religion dictates, we should find it in us to go past personal interests to fight self-serving tendencies in us. I hope what I shared with you, deeply personal as it is, will help you explore the facets in your own life, while always remembering to start with being kind to yourself, and those immediately around you. Seva starts at home!

Seva is a simple word. It means service. But I like to think of it in terms of togetherness with your community. When we dedicate ourselves to seva, not only are we devoting ourselves to God, whatever your concept of God may be, we are also giving ourselves the chance to live a longer, more satisfied, happier life.

~

- Shift focus away from yourself by doing seva for your community.
- Give your time and expertise for free to people who do not have the same privileges as you.
- Remind yourself every morning to be kind to yourself.
- Always do seva quietly, and expect nothing in return.

8

Staying Positive and Being Content

We have talked about asana, pranayama and dhyana. We have discussed in great detail what we should eat, drink and even how we should walk to help us live longer, more qualitatively better lives. But what about the power of the mind.

My grandfather used to say,

parāncikhāni vyatrnat svayambhūh
tasmāt parānpaśyati nāntarātmā |
kaściddīrah pratyagātmānamaiksat
āvrtta caksuh amratvan icchan||[1]

> The self-existent Lord pierced the openings [of the senses] outward; therefore one looks outward and not within oneself. Some wise person, however, desiring immortality, turned the gaze inward, and saw the indwelling Self.

By turning one's gaze inwards, we can ignore or simply sidestep the distractions around us. Introspection sounds like a heavy term, but think of how much control we can find through that. Instead of blaming the world around you when you think you have failed or are fearful, shouldn't we try and find control within us? But for that we first need to face and recognize that which is challenging to us.

Turn away from fear

Hear this story of a boy aged twelve who came to Mysore all alone. As he got off the train and started walking towards the King of Mysore's palace, he heard a very loud sound that stopped him in his tracks. Mysore was a big, foreign monster. He had never left home before. He was a scared and frightened little boy, dwarfed by the city, where everything was bigger than anything back home. And he almost turned around to go back to the train. But he didn't! Steeling himself he placed one foot ahead of the other and kept walking.

That boy was K. Pattabhi Jois. The year was 1927. And the loud sound was of the palace bells that tolled loudly every hour. This is the story I remember whenever I am faced with a challenging phase in my life.

When my grandfather came to Mysore to study at the Sanskrit College, he was so poor he couldn't afford any food. But he remained single-minded in his desire to be a scholar. My grandfather never lost hope. He went from house to house across Mysore to beg for food and that is how he sustained himself. He was lucky to come to the city in days when brahmacharyas were given a lot of respect.

Guruji always said studying was his first priority, and that was what gave him the strength to never lose focus on what he wanted to achieve. The family, him and then later his wife and children, truly saw days of poverty. They had no support. For years my grandmother only had two saris. That is all they could afford. My grandfather would tell me about days when his children had only one pair of clothes, so he would do extra work translating the Mahabharata and Ramayana in Kannada. There were very few books printed in Kannada those days, so Guruji would translate them from Sanskrit for people to read. He would get dakshina for that. Families would give him one dhoti (pancha) and that dhoti would be stitched as clothes for his children. Yet the family ploughed through. They didn't lose hope. They were content.

This is true yama niyama – to work honestly, without thinking of money or of cheating people to get ahead. When you work or live life in this manner, you will be happy with the results. You will be content, and that makes you peaceful.

Even if you aren't thinking about this during yoga, this should come naturally to you. Once you correct these fundamentals, then your family will follow suit.

If you survive in negativity that will multiply and will take over everything. The negativity of cheating people will grow inside you and make you unhappy. This was the mindset imbued in me as a child that I try to pass on to my children. An honest dedication to work.

I have seen many people come through the shala with all kinds of illnesses, even patients suffering from cancer. I know you will find this hard to believe, so did I at first, but a change in attitude helped them heal faster.

How does this translate into everyday life? You could be looking at a hard deadline, you may have a tough boss, a challenging relationship, attempting a tough Ashtanga posture or trying to complete a marathon. Through all of this our fears are but the rope in the Advaita story we learned about earlier. The snake is negativity, the fear of the unknown, but these are what prevent you from seeing other options, for you to see the snake is but a harmless rope, and your fears are unfounded.

When I come home to Mysore after travelling across bigger cities across the world, and drive on the streets here, I marvel at the lack of anger on the roads. People are kind and courteous, and everyone laughs in the face of chaos and a few scrapes here and there. What the small-town, laid-back citizens of Mysore lack in driving discipline, they make up in thoughtfulness, patience and magnanimity. And anyone who has driven in India will know how much of a challenge it can be. I don't know why this is so. Maybe it is because Mysore is home to the very sweet Mysore Pak? Or perhaps because it's the home of yoga in India, having been the birthplace of many great yogis from Guruji to T. Krishnamacharya and even B.K.S. Iyengar. I would like to think so, because that would make everything I live for worth it! I would love to translate the peacefulness of how Mysore lives into a lesson for life. I always tell my foreign students that is one of the factors that makes Mysore such a beautiful place to live in.

Have you ever stopped to think about what it takes to be magnanimous and kind in the face of stress? Everyone can be calm and loving when the going is good. But when your neighbour is fighting with you over a parking spot or someone is unfair at work, do you feel as kind?

Think of this mythological tale.

The Kauravas cheat the Pandavas by giving them barren land called Khandavaprastha. But the Pandavas work hard and transform it into Indraprastha. This is a simple, well-known, well-loved story. When faced with the difficulties life throws your way, when faced with challenges that come from within or outside you, this is what I ask you to look for within yourself – the ability to act maturely in the face of calamity, to see what we can do to create an Indraprastha out of every exacting situation or person.

The monkey in your mind

In Ashtanga we talk a lot about yamas. Instead of this being relegated to theory, I want us to try and see how we can channel ahimsa (non-violence) when we are feeling angry with others or with ourselves. When we get stressed about not getting a raise or fight for money, we can try and remember aparigraha (non-possessiveness). The monkey chatter that Buddha talked about is what makes us all push for more, faster, better, but what if we had a chat with that monkey during our meditation, reasoned with it, ask what is the point of the sacrifice of sleep, food and rest. And how this pressure affects us, our words and our actions.

In the Bhagavad Gita, Krishna says, 'Brooding on the objects of the senses, man develops attachment to them; attachment begets desire and from desire arises anger ... Anger then begets delusion, delusion befuddles the memory and confused memory corrupts reason. Thence arises total ruination.'[2] As scripted in every religious doctrine and philosophical conversation, most anxiety comes from objects of the senses. The Gita also compares a self-realized person to the undisturbed ocean into which many rivers flow. And goes on to compare such a person to one who is unhappy and greedy, for whom nothing is ever enough, whose desire of worldly objects produces only mental agitation, suffering and sorrow.

What does this mean? Desire causes disease of the mind and the body. Don't get me wrong. I think it's very important to have goals, and work towards them. Whatever our profession we all live by deadlines, and place a lot of stress on ourselves to achieve what we think are 'perfect' lives. If you carry negativity within you and crave for negative things, this will bring negativity to you.

If we can stop before lashing out, before reacting, would we find the world a better place to live in? Once we realize that the only thing we have control over is ourselves will this bring us closer to a perfect life?

These words highlight the importance of positive thinking, a practice that has become a big buzzword on shelves. But this isn't just self-help jargon.

There are two illnesses of the physical body, that which comes through lifestyle and that which is genetic. Yes, illness can be cured by medicine, but I continue to maintain that a permanent solution is only found with yogic practice.

Positivity leads to a happier and calm state of being and lowers the burden on our mind and body. Optimistic women have a significantly lower risk of dying from cancer, heart disease and stroke, among other causes.[3] There is a direct correlation between optimism and physical/mental well-being.[4] Optimistic people are more equipped to handle stress, since they are more resilient and have better coping strategies.

There are many ways in which we can make ourselves more inclined to positivity, and the most obvious is by doing something you enjoy, that fills you with joy. Just a few hours in a week with a loved one, or perhaps taking time out to play an instrument, write, paint, cook, meditate, exercise or practise Ashtanga Yoga, is all one needs to come back to the daily grind refreshed and with a more optimistic outlook. And we will see lowered depression and anxiety, better physical well-being and even a longer life!

Don't sacrifice happiness because there is a voice in your head which is telling you you're a failure, or making you fearful and anxious. Those are just snakes disguised as ropes. Don't face your problems with the same mindset that causes the problem.

How relationships can make us happy

Then there are your relationships. A Harvard study from 1938 found that people who were satisfied with their relationships at age 50 were the healthiest at age 80. This was a long-running test to see how people fared after a few decades. It found that more than money or fame, what helped to delay mental and physical decline was close and happy relationships. This gives you the tools to face the world with positivity. Which in turn helps you consider life from a space of calmness, and access a space of inner peace.

It is the strong bond we have with our family and samskara that teaches you to be strong, positive and honest. Children are sponges and the future of this world. So, set a good example for them. If schools can also impart these teachings, then slowly entire neighbourhoods and cities will change.

The best time to channel these energies is first thing in the morning! Even before you brush your teeth, clean your mind with positive thoughts. And yes, we can't stop negativity and that's why I recommend we recite a prayer or chant in the evenings and the mornings.

Ganesha – the remover of obstacles – is right in front of our beds, so that he is the first person we see when we wake up. Get up with happiness, otherwise your entire day is ruined. Wake up with love, positivity and contentment, instead of worrying about the things you don't have!

~

- Channel positivity first thing in the morning.
- Cure yourself of anxiety by searching inwards for contentment.
- Encourage honesty within your family and teach your children how to work and live with empathy and honesty.

Epilogue

Whatever one may to do to live a healthy, long life we can't escape death which is inevitable. Preparing for death is difficult and distressing. And we all pray for health and longevity of those around us and those we love. But there is another important aspect to this that I feel is very important, but which we choose to ignore, because it scares us – the idea that we can be prepared for death. Our own and that of those around us. According to Indian mythology, there are four stages in our lives, and we can prepare ourselves for death by making ourselves familiar with those stages.

Brahmacharya: This stage includes Balashrama, which is from before you hit puberty around fourteen continues till twenty-four. This is the stage when one gets educated and is taught the texts and mantra.

Brahmacharya also means celibacy. This represents the stage when you should concentrate on your studies and make yourself a better human being.

Grihastha: This is the stage to start a family. You get married, develop a relationship with your wife. This phase of your life is to focus on your family unit. At this stage you can no longer live as an island, and must devote yourself to your children and your partner. You do everything together. You stay together, you create a family. When you get married you take saptapadi – seven steps – you promise your future spouse you will help them during all difficulties, commit to each other. This is the understanding you make to your family. This stage is from twenty-five to sixty years.

Many sadhus skip this stage and jump into the next ashram. If you choose to have a family be close to your spouse and build a good understanding. When you choose to have children, it will then be your responsibility to ensure your children are educated and do well in their studies and become responsible citizens.

Vanaprastha: At this stage you start detaching. You hand over control of businesses to your children.

You become more spiritual. People at this stage start visiting places of worship. They start reading philosophies. You work towards leaving your physical body. You don't feel like earning too much money and don't want recognition at this stage. You have seen everything in the last stage.

You work to rid yourself of material attachments – you start to practise aparigraha, the Hindu virtue of non-possessiveness and non-greediness.

Sanyasa: In this stage, around the time you are seventy-five years old, you get ready to leave your body and your family. To work towards this, you break all worldly ties, you are no longer attached to anyone or any material possessions.

When the end comes you should want to leave the body smoothly. Your life should go from your body smoothly. Only then you will get moksha.

Notes

Introduction

1. Bhagavad Gita. Chapter 4, shloka 2.
2. Patanjali. *Yoga Sutra*. Chapter 1, sutra 14.

1. Eat Less to Live Longer

1. Svoboda, Robert. *Ayurveda Life Health and Longevity*. Ayurvedic Press, 1992.
2. 'Understanding of the vital source of life: agni (digestive fire)', Meenakshi Gupta, *Yoga Digest*. https://yogadigest.com/understanding-of-the-vital-source-of-life-agni-digestive-fire/
3. Bhagavad Gita. Chapter 6, shloka 17.
4. Ameneh Madjd, et al. 'Beneficial Effect of High Energy Intake at Lunch Rather Than Dinner on Weight Loss in Healthy Obese Women in a Weight-Loss Program:

a Randomized Clinical Trial', In *American Journal of Clinical Nutrition*. (2016).

5. Macdiarmid, Jennie. 'Seasonality and Dietary Requirements: Will Eating Seasonal Food Contribute to Health and Environmental Sustainability?' In *Proceedings of the Nutrition Society* 73, no. 3 (2014): 368–75.

6. Svoboda, Robert. *Ayurveda Life Health and Longevity*. Ayurvedic Press, 1992.

2. Eat Like a Yogi

1. Macdiarmid, Jennie. 'Seasonality and Dietary Requirements: Will Eating Seasonal Food Contribute to Health and Environmental Sustainability?' In *Proceedings of the Nutrition Society* 73, no. 3 (2014): 368–75.

2. Patel, Suchita, et al. 'Say Yes to Warm for Remove Harm: Amazing Wonders of Two Stages of Water!' In *European Journal of Medical and Pharmaceutical Research*.

3. Franke, A., et al. 'Postprandial Walking But Not Consumption of Alcoholic Digestifs or Espresso Accelerates Gastric Emptying in Healthy Volunteers.' In *Journal of Gastrointestinal and Liver Diseases* 17, no. 1 (2008): 27–31.

4. 'Really, the Claim Taking a Walk After a Meal Aids Digestion', *New York Times*, 24 June 2013.

3. How to Perfect Your Daily Routine

1. Benson, Herbert and Miriam J. Klipper. *The Relaxation Response.* HarperCollins, 1975.
2. Based on study conducted by Dr Andrew Newberg at Centre for Spirituality and the Mind at the University of Pennsylvania.
3. Benson, Herbert and Miriam J. Klipper. *The Relaxation Response*. HarperCollins, 1975.

4. Flood, Gavin. *The Ascetic Self: Subjectivity, Memory and Tradition*. Cambridge University Press, 2005.5.
   Sokal K. and P. Sokal. 'Earthing the Human Body Influences Physiologic Processes.' In *Journal of Alternative and Complementary Medicine* 17, no. 4 (2011): 301–308.
6. Akerstedt T., et al. 'Sleep Duration and Morality: Does Weekend Sleep Matter?' In *Journal of Sleep Research*. (2018).
7. 'Appetitive and Replacement Naps: EEG and Behaviour', F. Evans et al. *Science (New York)*, 1977.

4. Fast Once Every Fifteen Days

1. Genius, Stephen J., et al. 'Human Excretion of Bisphenol A: Blood, Urine, and Sweat (BUS) Study.' In *Journal of Environmental and Public Health*. (2012).
2. Ibid.

5. 10 Asanas are All You Need to Do

1. 'One Day in the Life of a Suffocating Planet – as it happened', Chris Michael, *Guardian*, 13 February 2017.
2. The Lancet Commission, 2015.
3. Savami Svatmarama. *Hatha Yoga Pradipika*.
4. Aditya Hridayam.
5. Jois, Pattabhi. *Yoga Mala*. India: Picador, 2010.

7. Help Others to Help Yourself

1. Umberson, Debra and Jennifer K. Montez. 'Social Relationships and Health: A Flashpoint for Health Policy.' In *Journal of Health and Social Behaviour*, no. 51 (2010).
2. Ryan, Richard M., et al. 'Vitalizing Effects of Being Outdoors and in Nature.' In *Journal of Environmental Psychology* 30, no. 2 (2010): 159–168.

8. Staying Positive

1. Kathopanishad, fourth valli, shloka 1.
2. Bhide, Ajit V. 'Anger and the Mahaabhaarata.' In *Indian Journal of Psychiatry* 49, no. 2 (2007): 140–142.
3. S. Eric et al. 'Optimism and Cause-Specific Mortality: A Prospective Cohort Study.' In *American Journal of Epidemology* 185, no. 1 (2017): 21–29.
4. Conversano, Ciro, et al. 'Optimism and Its Impact on Mental and Physical Well-Being.' In *Clinical Practice and Epidemiology in Mental Health* 6. (2010): 25–29.

Acknowledgements

I would like to thank my wife without whose support I would not be able to teach on such crazy schedules and my children, who fill my house with joy and love. My grand-mother and my mother who brought me up and taught me to love yoga.

And my students who also teach me something new every day.

A Note on the Authors

Sharath Jois is the grandson and student of the greatest Ashtanga master K. Pattabhi Jois who was responsible for making yoga popular the West. Sharath is the head of the Ashtanga Yoga Institute in Mysore, where thousands of students from around the world come to learn from him. Sharath was Pattabhi Jois's only student who has studied and continues to practise the complete six series of the Ashtanga Yoga system.

Isha Singh Sawhney, the co-author, lives in New Delhi with her cats and husband. She can be found making kombucha tea or practising Ashtanga Yoga when not working on her collection of short stories.

L

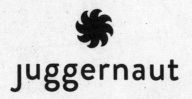

juggernaut

THE APP FOR INDIAN READERS

Fresh, original books tailored for mobile and for India. Starting at ₹10.

juggernaut.in

1

CRAFTED
FOR MOBILE
READING

Thought you would never read a book
on mobile? Let us prove you wrong.

A Note on the Authors

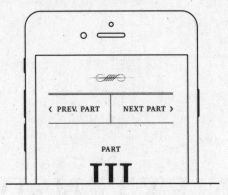

Beautiful Typography

The quality of print transferred to your mobile. Forget ugly PDFs.

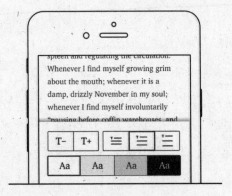

Customizable Reading

Read in the font size, spacing and background of your liking.

2

AN EXTENSIVE LIBRARY

Including fresh, new, original Juggernaut books from the likes of Sunny Leone, Praveen Swami, Husain Haqqani, Umera Ahmed, Rujuta Diwekar and lots more. Plus, books from partner publishers and loads of free classics. Whichever genre you like, there's a book waiting for you.

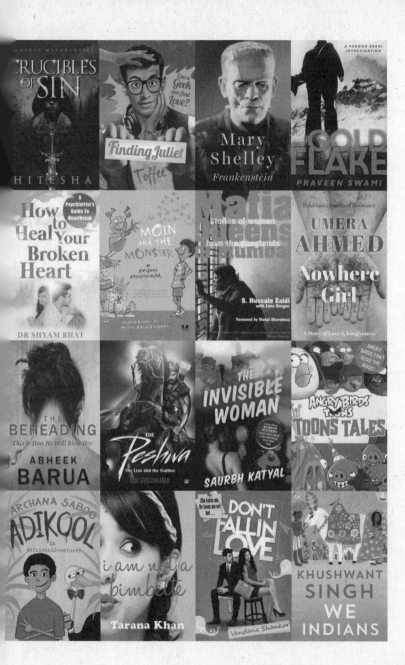

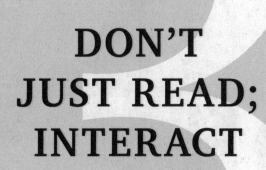

DON'T JUST READ; INTERACT

We're changing the reading experience from passive to active.

Ask authors questions

Get all your answers from the horse's mouth.
Juggernaut authors actually reply to every
question they can.

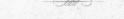

Rate and review

Let everyone know of your favourite reads or
critique the finer points of a book – you will be
heard in a community of like-minded readers.

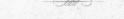

Gift books to friends

For a book-lover, there's no nicer gift than
a book personally picked. You can even
do it anonymously if you like.

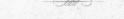

Enjoy new book formats

Discover serials released in parts over
time, picture books including comics,
and story-bundles at discounted rates.
And coming soon, audiobooks.

4

LOWEST PRICES & ONE-TAP BUYING

Books start at ₹10 with regular discounts and free previews.

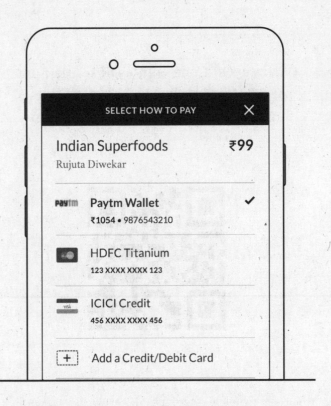

SELECT HOW TO PAY ✕

Indian Superfoods ₹99
Rujuta Diwekar

Paytm Wallet ✓
₹1054 • 9876543210

HDFC Titanium
123 XXXX XXXX 123

ICICI Credit
456 XXXX XXXX 456

+ Add a Credit/Debit Card

Paytm Wallet, Cards & Apple Payments

On Android, just add a Paytm Wallet once and buy any book with one tap. On iOS, pay with one tap with your iTunes-linked debit/credit card.

Click the QR Code with a QR scanner app
or type the link into the Internet browser
on your phone to download the app.

For our complete catalogue, visit www.juggernaut.in
To submit your book, send a synopsis and two
sample chapters to books@juggernaut.in
For all other queries, write to contact@juggernaut.in